Praise for Telling Tales About Dementia

'These personal accounts by family carers, harrowing, distressing, but also inspiring and uplifting, will have you weeping one moment and laughing the next, as they describe struggling to manage situations that range from horrific to comical. How do you cope alone with your loved one's slow loss of rational thought and behaviour? You cannot – and you need not. The single most valuable achievement of this book is to tell carers they are not alone. The more of us there are, the stronger we become, and the better we can fight for our loved ones in the face of this cruel disease.'

– John Suchet, broadcaster and Patron of for dementia, *who is caring for his wife, Bonnie, who has dementia*

'These accounts are a tribute to the abiding insistence on according dignity to every one of us until our last breath. Reading these stories will make us all, in the words of one of the contributors, "determined to make a difference".'

– fr

'This anthology of carers' stories possesses the of emotion. The honest accounts of families ca with dementia are inspiring, uplifting and yet at times heart-wrenchingly tragic. It is a captivating and essential read for all professionals trying to understand and help families caring for a loved one living with dementia. Echoes of indifference in the face of family devotion and upset stand in distressingly sharp contrast. I was left in no doubt that all health and social care practitioners, including those working in care homes, who read these tales will be unable to stop themselves looking at what they do and asking can we not do better?'

– Dr Graham Stokes, Consultant Clinical Psychologist and Head of Psychology Services for Older People at South Staffordshire and Shropshire Healthcare NHS Foundation Trust, Head of Mental Health at Bupa Care Homes, and author of And Still the Music Plays: Stories of People with Dementia *(Hawker Books 2008)*

'These powerful stories should be read by everyone involved in health and social care, from commissioners designing services to those giving direct care and support. I hope they will also be read by those who have had no previous contact with dementia, to help combat the stigma it still carries through lack of public awareness.

The accounts are moving, engrossing, sprinkled with quirky humour, and truthful. There is both warm praise and angry criticism of services. I hope the book will play its part alongside the National Dementia Strategy to help eradicate some of the glaring bad practice it highlights.

Vivid personalities shine through, reminding us that every person with dementia, every carer and every caring relationship is different and individual, therefore services need to be sensitive, personal and flexible.'

– Sue Benson, Editor of The Journal of Dementia Care

'The stories of these carers – sisters, brothers, husbands, wives, lovers and friends – are not confined to the painful subject of dementia: the book is also about anger, loss, love and loyalty. It's both powerful and moving.'

– Diana Melly, writer and widow of jazz legend, George
Melly, who had dementia in his final years

Telling
Tales
About
Dementia

of related interest

Losing Clive to Younger Onset Dementia
One Family's Story
Helen Beaumont
ISBN 978 1 84310 480 3

Dancing with Dementia
My Story of Living Positively with Dementia
Christine Bryden
ISBN 978 1 84310 332 5

A Personal Guide to Living with Progressive Memory Loss
Sandy Burgener and Prudence Twigg
ISBN 978 1 84310 863 4

Alzheimer
A Journey Together
Federica Caracciolo
Foreword by Luisa Bartorelli
ISBN 978 1 84310 408 7

Telling Tales About Dementia

Experiences of Caring

EDITED BY LUCY WHITMAN

FOREWORD BY JOANNA TROLLOPE

Jessica Kingsley Publishers
London and Philadelphia

First published in 2010
by Jessica Kingsley Publishers
116 Pentonville Road
London N1 9JB, UK
and
400 Market Street, Suite 400
Philadelphia, PA 19106, USA

www.jkp.com

Library of Congress Cataloging in Publication Data
Telling tales about dementia : carers share their stories / edited by Lucy Whitman ; foreword
by Joanna Trollope.
   p. cm.
 ISBN 978-1-84310-941-9 (alk. paper)
 1. Dementia--Patients--Care. 2. Caregivers' writings, American. I. Whitman, Lucy, 1954-
 RC521.T45 2009
 616.8'3--dc22
                                   2009010543

British Library Cataloguing in Publication Data
A CIP catalogue record for this book is available from the British Library

ISBN 978 1 84310 941 9

Printed and bound in Great Britain by
Athenaeum Press, Gateshead, Tyne and Wear

Contents

Living with Loss

Despatches from the Battlefield

Keeping in Touch, Letting Go

Foreword

Joanna Trollope OBE, Patron, **for dementia**

My father was born in 1914, and lived until he was 89. You might say that 89 was a very good innings, except for the fact that almost all of the last fifteen of those 89 years were clouded by his increasing dementia. And, like so many of the cases described in this remarkable collection, it was not a tranquil dementia. As so often chronicled here, his illness affected the whole family acutely, especially – and obviously – my mother. The whole miserable business was made worse, I'm afraid, by lack of clarity in diagnosis, by a persistent social reluctance to acknowledge the illness, and an

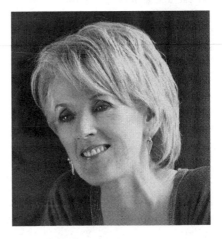

Joanna Trollope © Barker Evans

absence of proper support. And I'm only talking about under a decade ago.

This book will come as an immense relief to the thousands of people whose lives are affected by this cruel condition – and it also comes at a time of change. Dementia is, at last, being publicly admitted and seriously medically addressed. The invaluable work of Admiral nurses in alleviating patients' distress, and helping their family carers not to go clean round the bend with the strain of looking after them, is finally being publicised, celebrated and – I do hope – increased. With all of us living longer, and facing the real possibility of outliving our own sanity, we need all the research and assistance we can get.

The profile of dementia, in all its forms, has of course been sharply raised by the extraordinary courage and candour shown by well-known people such as Terry Pratchett, who has Alzheimer's, and John Suchet, whose wife suffers from dementia. But what this book demonstrates, just as eloquently and bravely, is the astonishing stoicism, persistence and good humour of private people dealing with the dementia of their families and friends.

They battle with social stigma, indifference, violence, squalor, medical incompetence, homophobia, callousness, exhaustion, incontinence, loneliness, grief and unbelievable levels of frustration. Many of them also struggle to protect the rest of the family from the dementia, and with money worries. But despite all this wretchedness, as you will discover, there is an amazing resilience of spirit as well as a robust humour and a refusal to stop loving someone who has been grossly distorted by something he or she cannot help. These accounts are a tribute to the abiding insistence on according dignity to every one of us until our last breath. Reading these stories will make us all, in the words of one of the contributors, Maria Smith, 'determined to make a difference'.

March 2009

Preface

Barbara Stephens, Chief Executive, **for dementia**

for dementia
training ▪ development ▪ admiral nurses

for dementia welcomes this anthology, written by people from diverse backgrounds who have cared for someone with dementia.

Dementia has the potential to touch all our lives, either directly or indirectly. How important it is, therefore, that we take notice of those who know first-hand about this life-changing illness. We have so much to learn.

Telling Tales About Dementia reveals the true impact of dementia on people's lives. The stories told here are both moving and inspiring. They vividly reflect the tragedy of dementia, the gravity of loss and the complexity of the journey. Family carers also describe the frustration and despair they feel when battling with a system of health and social care which too often fails to look after us.

But there is hope and optimism too: clear indications that the quality of people's lives can be enhanced by sensitive and well-managed support services, by improved understanding of the impact of dementia on all those who are affected, and by recognising the importance of valuing all of us as human beings, and embracing and sustaining the connections between us.

This book will contribute, in a very significant way, to improving the knowledge of professionals working in the field. It will have the effect of raising awareness amongst those who are prepared to face this issue. Most importantly, it will provide a sense of affirmation for people currently affected by dementia, and for those who have waved it goodbye, but for whom its legacy lives on.

Acknowledgements

Lucy Whitman

I am very grateful for all the help, support and encouragement I have received in the preparation of this book. I particularly wish to thank:

Jules Jones, who first of all supported my family as our Admiral nurse. She showed an interest in the anthology at an early stage and introduced me to her colleagues at *for dementia*. Barbara Stephens, chief executive of *for dementia*, immediately gave the book her backing, and Joy Watkins, resource coordinator for Uniting Carers for Dementia, introduced me to many of the carers who have contributed to the anthology, and has continued to give me generous support throughout.

Staff at Alzheimer's Society have been extremely helpful, above all Janet Baylis, manager of the Dementia Knowledge Centre, who welcomed me into the cramped confines of the library at the old Alzheimer's Society headquarters (before they moved into their new premises) and made many thoughtful suggestions. The Alzheimer's Society website has been an invaluable source of information.

Staff at the Down's Syndrome Association kindly put me in touch with Peggy Fray. Gail Chester gave me the benefit of her experience as a seasoned anthology editor. Nancy Croft has listened to every detail of the project as it unfolded. My editor at Jessica Kingsley Publishers, Helen Ibbotson, has been very supportive. Special thanks to U Hla Htay for permission to use the photo on the cover, and to all the contributors who supplied photos of themselves and the people they have cared for. Thanks also to Mavis Pilbeam for tireless proofreading.

Friends, colleagues and acquaintances have all shown an interest and in many cases either contributed to the book, introduced me to other potential contributors, offered feedback on draft material or helped in other ways. Thanks very much to: Jaye Akintola, Brian Baylis, Abul Choudhury, Rosemary Clarke, Russell Clifton, Rosemary Cox, Tim Dartington, Rachael Dixey, Sandra Evans, Lenny Fagin, Andrea Gover, Maria Jastrzębska, Sophie Laws, Graham Lock, Geraldine McCarthy, Natalie Morris, Roger Newman, Shirley Nurock, Barbara Ongley, Nicky Parker, Zimena Percival, Julie-Ann Phillips, Maggie Playle, Neill Quinton, Ruth Robinson, John Rousell, Mick Scully, Ralph Smith, Rhonda Smith, Mohammed Subhan, Rachel Thompson.

Thanks also to my family, especially my son Ben who is such a good companion, and my sister Rosalind who gave me much-appreciated help at a critical time.

Above all, of course, I am indebted to all the contributors who have told their tales in this book, and shared their experiences for the benefit of others. It has been an enriching experience for me to collaborate with them in creating this anthology.

This book is dedicated to the memory of my parents Elizabeth and George Whitman.

*I*ntroduction

Lucy Whitman

Who the book is for

First and foremost, this book is for people who are caring for someone with dementia, or who have done so in the past. I hope it will provide comfort and reassurance – you are not alone. Other people have trodden this path before you. Second, I hope that members of the general public will be interested. You may not be affected by dementia today, but perhaps tomorrow you will be. Finally, I sincerely hope that health and social service professionals, whether or not they specialise in dementia care, will read the book, and that it will contribute to greater awareness within these professions about the needs of people with dementia and those who care for them.

Dementia – a bewildering condition

I know now that my biggest difficulty was the fact that I knew nothing about dementia. I didn't even know the word, and, worse still, simply thought my mother was 'going senile' as her mother had done, and that we just had to do the best we could. The district nurse from her GP practice didn't mention the word, didn't mention diagnosis, didn't mention memory clinics or drugs for dementia, or the Alzheimer's Society or support groups or respite care… As far as I knew, I just had to get on with it and do the best I could, and we lurched together into what became a kind of awful chaos. (Rosemary Clarke, 'State of Grace')

Like Rosemary and many of the other contributors to this book, my family stumbled without knowledge or guidance into this 'awful chaos' when my mother developed dementia in the last years of her life. It is terrible to lose someone you love to any terminal illness, but dementia is a bewildering condition, both for the person whose brain is under attack, and for his or her relatives and friends.

All those who care for a sick or disabled person have to make enormous physical and emotional efforts, have to manage a calendar of appointments with countless health and social care professionals, have to fight to make sure the person they are caring for receives all the benefits and support to which he or she is entitled, have to manage somehow to fit their caring tasks around their other commitments, such as work and family. But looking after someone with dementia has an additional, surreal quality to it.

Dementia is associated with memory loss, but in many cases this is not the first or even the most obvious symptom. The first sign that something is amiss may be that a person you know very well starts behaving in a strange way, becoming unaccountably suspicious/anxious/timid/aggressive/obsessive/generally 'unreasonable'. Individuals may make misjudgements in their financial affairs, or start to drive erratically, and yet be apparently unaware that they are putting themselves and others at risk.

Most of us go into denial at this stage: This can't really be happening. It's just a one-off, a 'senior moment', a bad patch. Surely they could remember/ understand/drive more carefully if they tried just a bit harder? Many of us also encounter institutional denial, from GPs, psychiatrists, hospital staff. 'It's just stress.' 'It's just depression.' 'She's just a bit confused.' 'It's just his age.' 'It's nothing to worry about.'

Communication becomes difficult. The carer becomes weary and irritable at having to answer the same questions over and over again. Conversations become strange. 'And what do you think about this idea they've got, of trying to get me to have another baby?' my 90-year-old mother exclaimed. 'I must be losing my bonkers!' announced Steve Jeffery's mother ('A Very Important Moustache'). Eventually, language itself is lost.

It is chilling when your mother, who brought you into the world, or your partner with whom you have shared the last 30 years, no longer recognises you. The ground seems to shift beneath your feet. It is deeply unnerving, and strikes at the carer's own sense of self as well as that of the person with dementia.

The lack of knowledge, and the bewilderment felt both by people with dementia and their carers is mirrored in the widespread ignorance and confusion about this condition which has permeated our health and social services up to the present date, and which is amply illustrated in the chapters which follow.

However, there is reason to hope that this may now begin to change for the better. In February 2009, the Department of Health published its National Dementia Strategy for England, *Living Well with Dementia* (to be followed by strategies for the other nations of the UK). The strategy sets out ambitious plans to improve all aspects of dementia care, and starts with the recognition that raising awareness about dementia, both amongst the general public and the medical profession, must be a top priority if we are to improve the lives of those who are affected.[1]

At present, most people with dementia never receive a formal diagnosis or have contact with specialist services at any time in their illness.[2] Without a diagnosis, there can be no appropriate treatment and support. Support does exist, but many people with dementia and their carers do not ask for help until the situation is desperate. By this time, in the words of the National Dementia Strategy:

> opportunities for harm prevention and maximisation of quality of life have passed. If dementia is not diagnosed, the person with dementia and their family carers are denied the possibility of making choices themselves. They are unable to make informed plans for their future and do not have access to the help, support and treatments...which can help.[3]

It would have made such a difference, to my own family and to many of the families which feature in this book, if we had been offered information, advice and support at an early stage, rather than being left to struggle on as best we could, trying to make sense of a baffling situation.

What is dementia?

The National Dementia Strategy defines dementia as follows:

> The term 'dementia' is used to describe a syndrome which may be caused by a number of illnesses in which there is progressive decline in multiple areas of function, including decline in memory, reasoning, communication skills and the ability to carry out daily activities. Alongside this decline, individuals may develop behavioural and psychological symptoms such as depression, psychosis, aggression and wandering, which complicate care and which can occur at any stage of the illness.[4]

The most common types of dementia are Alzheimer's disease and vascular dementia (sometimes known as multi-infarct dementia). Rarer types of dementia include dementia with Lewy bodies and fronto-temporal dementia.

All these diseases are progressive (they will get worse over time), and terminal (they will eventually lead to death).

Research carried out for the Alzheimer's Society's Dementia UK Report suggests that there are nearly 700,000 people with dementia in the UK (more than 1% of the population), and that this number will probably double within the next 30 years.[5] It is possible to develop dementia at any age, but the likelihood increases with age. One in 50 people between the ages of 65 and 70 has some form of dementia, compared to one in five people over 80.[6]

What is a carer?

The organisation Carers UK defines carers as people who 'provide unpaid care by looking after an ill, frail or disabled family member, friend or partner'.[7]

For the purposes of this book, the term 'carer' is used somewhat more broadly. It refers to anyone who is in a close personal relationship with the person who has dementia, and, in most cases, takes on the responsibility of making sure that the person with dementia is safe and well looked after. The carer may share a home with the person with dementia, and may be doing the 'hands on' caring, including all the washing and feeding, heavy lifting and laundry; or he or she may be organising professional care, managing the practical arrangements and doing a lot of worrying, perhaps from a distance. The term 'carer' can also include other family members or friends who have been profoundly affected because someone they *care about* has developed dementia. This includes the children growing up in a home where one parent has dementia, such as the Malik family ('Our Mum Had To Be the Man of the House'), or the grown-up son or daughter travelling home regularly to support their mother, who is caring for her husband, such as Ian McQueen ('Family Matters').

Many people fall into the role of carer in a gradual and imperceptible way, and do not recognise the term when it is first applied to them. 'The practice counsellor told me that I was a carer,' writes Andra Houchen ('Strained to the Limit'). 'I had no idea what this meant. As far as I knew I was a wife, a mother, going out to work, trying to help my husband who was ill in some unfathomable way, and doing my best to help him through this depression, bad patch or mid-life crisis.'

How this book came into being

When I was caring for my mother, I did not have time to join a carers' support group, but I did read some books about dementia, to try to get a grip on the situation. I found myself riveted, appalled, comforted and tantalised by the snippets of people's real life experiences which appear in the various introductory guides to dementia. Some years after my mother's death, I knew I needed to write about my experience, and it occurred to me that a collection of different people's experiences would be useful to others in a similar situation. Possible contributors were identified by approaches to various carers' organisations, notably Uniting Carers for Dementia, as well as friends, colleagues and acquaintances. Dementia is so widespread that almost everyone I spoke to about the book wanted to tell me about someone they knew. I solicited contributions from a wide range of people, but the resulting book is not a scientific sample; no single volume could be comprehensive, or completely representative.

The book is divided into three main sections, Living with Loss, Despatches from the Battlefield and Keeping in Touch, Letting Go.

Living with Loss

In the first part of the book, people from different backgrounds and in different circumstances describe the grief of losing a loved parent or partner to dementia.

Maria Jastrzębska, whose family came to England from Poland after the war, Debbie Jackson who fled apartheid South Africa with her husband, U Hla Htay from Burma, Maria Smith from Italy, Geraldine McCarthy from Ireland, all describe the heartbreak of seeing loved ones transformed before their eyes.

There is the utter shock of learning that your partner, with whom you were looking forward to a happy retirement, has developed an incurable, progressive brain disease. 'I *still* find it hard to believe that Alzheimer's has happened to *us*,' writes Rachael Dixey ('Walking on Thin Ice'), 'as if we were sent the wrong script.'

Certain dates are never to be forgotten: the day the diagnosis was given, the day the person you love went to live in a care home.

As well as the grief and shock, there is the stress and exhaustion, the relentless pressure and the sheer hard work that caring entails. On top of the daily grind, there are the regular crises – another fall, another infection, another hospital admission, more often than not leading to a further deterioration in the condition of the person you are caring for. Recent research appears to confirm what many of us have long suspected – that falls, infections and major surgery may all accelerate cognitive decline.[8]

There is enormous compassion and tenderness, but also frustration and sometimes resentment – and, inevitably, guilt. There is also the longing to escape. 'Today when I woke up I wanted to be somewhere else. But as usual, I will struggle with the wheelchair again, pushing and shoving it into the boot of the car, along with the seat, the bag, the hat and gloves, the nappy bag with spare pads and wipes, and go and collect him from the home' (Anna Young, 'Half a World Away').

Dementia inhibits communication with those we are caring for, but within the world of dementia care we make new connections, with kindly doctors and nurses and volunteers, with other carers who are 'in the same boat' and know what we are going through, with the army of paid careworkers who have come from all over the world to help us look after our frail relations – often leaving their own children or ageing parents behind. 'What they saved, they sent home to the families they'd had to leave behind in order to provide for them by working abroad. This was particularly poignant when one of the carers lost her own mother during her time with us.' (Maria Jastrzębska, 'A Big Enough Supply of Love').

Despatches from the Battlefield

Some people with dementia and their families receive excellent care and support, but sadly this is not always the case. The second section of the book focuses on instances where the pain of losing someone we care about to dementia is exacerbated by failings in the services which are meant to help us.

Many contributors voice their anger at the neglect and indignities suffered by their parents or partners in hospitals or care homes. Habitual practices which service providers apparently regard as unimportant – such as male carers assisting women in the toilet, patients left half-naked in a mixed ward, or residents appearing in other people's clothes – all of these practices absolutely enrage family carers, for they reveal a failure to recognise the person with dementia as worthy of respect and even common courtesy.

'The indignity of being in a care home where Dad would so often appear in other people's clothes, and thus lose so much more of his identity through no fault of his own, was heartbreaking for all of us,' writes Rosie Smith ('Forever in my Thoughts'). Why is it so hard for care homes to ensure all clothing is returned to its rightful owner after being washed? How would the care home owner like to be dressed in someone else's ill-fitting clothes?

Unexplained bruises, teeth not cleaned and left to decay, pressure sores being allowed to develop unchecked, food or medicine being left on the bedside table out of reach, dehydration and malnutrition because staff do not take the time to feed the people in their care, frightened patients on hospital wards crying out for help, but ignored by the nurses who regard them as a 'nuisance' – these are just some of the situations which give family carers sleepless nights.

Dementia is seen as an illness of old age. Our society does not, in general, cherish or value old people, and this is probably why inadequate attention and resources are devoted to dementia care, treatment and research. But the institutional ageism which consigns many older people with dementia to neglect and indignity does not mean that younger people with dementia get a better deal. Far from it. Dementia is a cruel illness at whatever age it strikes, but for those who develop dementia at an early age, and for their families, there is additional anguish.

In many parts of the country, the only services for people with dementia that exist have been designed with frail elderly people in mind; they are often quite unsuitable for younger people who may be physically fit and energetic, and may be displaying what is euphemistically termed 'challenging behaviour'. Indeed, many care homes and day centres are not even licensed to accept clients under 65. Pat Brown's chapter, 'Cracks in the System', charts a nightmare journey through an illogical and uncaring system. Her family encountered careworkers, psychiatrists and social workers who had no awareness of the behaviour or needs of people with dementia, and her husband was subjected to terrifying assessment procedures, which only served to aggravate his volatile condition.

It has been estimated that about 18,000 people throughout the UK are living with younger onset dementia, defined as dementia which develops before the age of 65.[9] This may be an underestimate, since GPs and even psychiatrists do not always recognise it. Both Pat Brown and Andra Houchen ('Strained to the Limit') suffered for years, along with their children, because their husbands' dementia was misdiagnosed as depression. When anti-depressants did not work, Andra Houchen's husband was subjected to electro-convulsive therapy (ECT). The psychologist who assessed Pat Brown's husband refused to believe the evidence of his own tests, and concluded that Chris Brown was 'putting it on' in order to secure early retirement.

The biggest problem for Andra Houchen was that neither the GP nor the various psychiatrists who examined her husband would listen to what she had to tell them. Her husband's behaviour became increasingly bizarre, but he resolutely refused to admit there was anything wrong with him. The doctors insisted that they could not discuss her husband's case with her, on grounds of 'patient confidentiality'.

Patient confidentiality is a fine ideal, but when dementia is, or may be, part of the equation, a rigid adherence to this principle may actually act against the interests of the patient. If patients themselves are unable to recognise that there is a problem, or are unable to speak on their own behalf, they may miss out on vital treatment and care. (The people around them may also be forced to live, as Andra Houchen's family were, with 'inexplicable personality and character changes unaided', even though this drove Andra and her daughters to the brink of mental collapse themselves.) The National Dementia Strategy has identified the need for early diagnosis of dementia.[10] At present, early diagnosis is sometimes prevented by the refusal of doctors to listen to the people who know the patient best.

Brian Baylis ('The Significant Other') was also fobbed off on grounds of 'patient confidentiality', when, after years of acting as devoted carer and advocate for his friend Timothy – who was profoundly disabled by dementia and unable to voice his own wishes – he was suddenly excluded by social services from all further involvement. In this case, it would appear that homophobia (either conscious or unconscious) was at work. In Roger Newman's chapter, 'Surely the World has Changed?', he explains how the specific needs of lesbians and gay men affected by dementia are not always recognised or met by conventional services, and describes how he came to co-found the now thriving Alzheimer's Society LGBT (lesbian, gay, bisexual and transgender) carers' group.

People with Down's syndrome are at risk of developing Alzheimer's disease at a much earlier age than the rest of the population.[11] In 'A Sister's Story', Peggy Fray gives a moving account of how Alzheimer's stripped her sister Kathleen of her 'hard-won capabilities', and of how she battled against a system in which most care-providers had no experience or training in caring for people with this dual disability.

Gail Chester ('An Instruction Manual for Keeping your Mind') reports from another battlefield – that of her own mind: exploring the often unspoken fear of inheriting Alzheimer's.

Keeping in Touch, Letting Go

The final section of the book explores some of the ways carers have found to stay in close communication with someone at an advanced stage of dementia, when verbal language has been lost, and how they kept their partner or parent company as he or she journeyed towards death.

Tim Dartington ('The End of the Story') makes the point that most of us would like to die at home, but that at present this is quite hard to achieve. When people in the final stages of dementia contract an infection, or experience breathing problems, they are often whisked off to hospital by the emergency services, and may die there in unfamiliar and possibly frightening surroundings. With enormous determination, good professional support, a certain amount of planning and quite a lot of luck, Tim Dartington, Barbara

Pointon and Rosemary Clarke all succeeded in ensuring that the person they were caring for died in familiar surroundings, in the company of those who loved them.

Even at 'the end of the story', institutional denial rears its head. Tim Dartington concludes his account with the following words:

> The doctor gave the cause of death on the certificate as dementia – which was true enough. Strangely, the coroner's office would not accept so straight-forward an explanation and a new certificate had to be issued. Even in death there was a wish to find another explanation for what had been happening. (Tim Dartington, 'The End of the Story')

The challenge ahead

The National Dementia Strategy points out that the UK falls far behind its European neighbours, such as France, Ireland and Spain, with regard to the diagnosis and treatment of people with dementia.[12] Until now, dementia research, treatment and care has not been given the priority it deserves in the UK, given the large numbers of people affected.

But change is in the air. The government has finally recognised that it will cost more in the long run to go on ignoring dementia, and failing people with dementia and their families, than to invest in planned support. The National Dementia Strategy offers real hope that things can and will improve. The three principal aims of the strategy are: improved awareness and understanding of dementia; earlier diagnosis and intervention; and a higher quality of care and support for people living and dying with dementia.

In order to secure genuine, sustained improvements in the quality of life for people with dementia and their carers, however, there needs to be a massive, well-targeted investment of cash. In addition to the cost of setting up the specialist diagnostic and support services and the training schemes envisaged in the National Dementia Strategy, money is needed for all of the following:

- to end the anomaly whereby people with dementia usually have to fund their own care while those with other terminal illnesses receive free care[13]

- to increase the budget per head for the care of people with dementia, so that all are provided with high-quality person-centred care[14]

- to raise the pay of home care and residential careworkers to a decent level

- to raise the value of Carers' Allowance from its present paltry rate.

This anthology appears at a critical moment, soon after the publication of the National Dementia Strategy, and the stories in this book demonstrate the scope of the challenge ahead. Many of the testimonies vividly illustrate the serious failings within the current system, which the National Dementia Strategy sets out to rectify. I look forward to the time when we can look back on the horror stories recounted in Despatches from the Battlefield as a thing of the past.

Love stories with a difference

Working on this anthology has been an inspiring and uplifting experience. The stories in this book are an incredible testament to the power of love, love that endures 'in sickness and in health', 'till death us do part'.

It is noticeable that a high proportion of the contributors to this book are involved as volunteers in carers' support groups or campaigns, even if their own 'caring days' are over. There is something about caring for someone with dementia which changes you, and many carers and ex-carers feel the need to spread the word: to share what they have learned with others who are just starting out on this journey, or to campaign fiercely for improvements to services.

Maria Smith captures this impulse in her poem 'Feisty Love':

Only my spirit bounces against the hard rock of despair
and rises
each morning
to face the new day,
determined to make a difference.

Notes

[1]   Department of Health (2009) *Living Well with Dementia: A National Dementia Strategy*. London: Department of Health, pp.23–30. Available at www.dh.gov. uk/en/Publicationsandstatistics/Publications/PublicationsPolicyAndGuidance/ DH_094058, accessed 18 March 2009.

[2]   *Living Well with Dementia*, p.33.

[3]   *Living Well with Dementia*, p.17.

[4]   *Living Well with Dementia*, p.15.

[5]   Alzheimer's Society (2007) *Dementia UK*. London: Alzheimer's Society, p.xiv. Available at www.alzheimers.org.uk/downloads/Dementia_UK_Full_Report. pdf, accessed 6 May 2009.

6   Alzheimer's Society (2008) *Factsheet 450: Am I at Risk of Developing Dementia?* London: Alzheimer's Society. Available at www.alzheimers.org.uk/factsheet/450, accessed 18 March 2009.

7   Carers UK website, www.carersuk.org/Aboutus, accessed 18 March 2009.

8   Wellcome Trust Press Release 17 September 2008, 'Inflammatory response to infection and injury may worsen dementia' accessed 20 January 2009 at www. wellcome.ac.uk/News/Media-office/Press-releases/2008/WTX050472.htm referencing research by Dr Colm Cunningham (Trinity College Dublin) and colleagues. Cunningham, C., Campion, S., Lunnon, K., Murray, C., *et al.* (2009) 'Systematic inflammation induces acute behavioural and cognitive changes and accelerates neurodegenerative disease.' *Biological Psychiatry 65*, 4, 304–312, available online at http://dx.doi.org/doi:10.1016/j.biopsych.2008.07.024, accessed 6 May 2009.

9   Harvey, R., Skelton-Robinson, M. and Rossor, M.N. (2003) 'The prevalence and causes of dementia in people under the age of 65 years.' *Journal of Neurology, Neurosurgery and Psychiatry 74*, 1206–1209. Available at http://jnnp.bmj.com/cgi/content/full/74/9/1206, accessed 19 March 2009.

10   *Living Well with Dementia*, pp.31–38.

11   Holland, T. (2004) *Down's Syndrome and Alzheimer's Disease: A Guide for Parents and Carers.* Teddington: Down's Syndrome Association. Available at www.downs-syndrome.org.uk/resources/publications/medical-and-health.html, accessed 19 March 2009.

12   *Living Well with Dementia*, p.17.

13   Alzheimer's Society (2008) *The Dementia Tax.* London: Alzheimer's Society, p.xiv. Available at www.alzheimers.org.uk/site/scripts/download_info.php?downloadID=109&fileID= 411

14   *The Dementia Tax*, p.xv.

LIVING WITH LOSS

1

$\mathcal{A}$ Big Enough Supply of Love

Maria Jastrzębska

On the morning of my fiftieth birthday, like a child, I want to hear my parents' voices. I phone their house and their live-in carer answers and puts each of them in turn on the phone to me. Experience has taught me that if I ask my father to get my mother he forgets and I'm left dangling for ages, and my mother is physically unable either to fetch him or pass him the phone. I tell my father that it's my birthday and he wishes me many happy returns but is worried he didn't remember, so I reassure him that I will be coming up to London next week and it is all arranged for us to party together. My mother is less surprised by my announcement, but asks me how my horse is. It is one of those innumerable situations when I can either go along with her, and tell her my horse is doing very well indeed thank you, or try to get to the bottom of what she means by my horse, given that I live in a semi in Hove and neither possess nor ride any horses. Perhaps she means one of our cats, perhaps my partner Deborah or my daughter Elena – or perhaps she really thinks I have a horse. Both my parents had dementia, and this is a typical snapshot of my communication with them at that time.

Nowadays when friends tell me their parents are no longer able to look after themselves, I want to laugh – not unkindly, but with the mild hysteria of familiarity. Sure enough, the next thing they say, with a puzzled or hurt expression, is that these same parents keep rejecting the very good help which they are at great pains to set up for them. And I can't help wondering whether, when the time comes, I would accept help graciously or not.

My father was the first to develop dementia. If dementia can ever be called gentle, my father's began almost gently with the loss of his short-term memory, the result of minor strokes. My mother became his primary carer which eventually took its toll on her own health. During a period when she was staying in the local rehabilitation hospital for the elderly, I enlisted the support of a kind and wise Polish nun to persuade my mother to take on some care when she returned home. Though not religious myself, I found my parents' local Polish church to be one of the places where support for them was forthcoming. For a few weeks it seemed to work, but one weekend I went away and came back to find my mother had got rid of the new carers. She complained that the carers were useless and lazy, and they complained that she wouldn't let them do anything. We were back to square one. Meanwhile, my father's memory was deteriorating. He would forget to turn off the gas and become easily disorientated. He could not remember whether he had eaten a meal and/or taken his anticoagulant medication.

The onset of my mother's dementia took a much more dramatic form. She had had a series of falls. No one realised that she had in fact fractured her hip. It was one of those fractures which are difficult to detect, and I can't help remembering that I was encouraging her to exercise, thinking her pain was arthritic. Finally, she was admitted to hospital and had emergency surgery and the shock of it, on top of Parkinson's, which she had been diagnosed with a couple of years before, tipped her over the edge. I was visiting her and caring for my father twice a week, coming up from Brighton to London, and she would tell me that the hospital was on fire and could I please do something to get her out.

She'd never been an easy woman. Like many people who had lived through the Nazi occupation, followed by a decade of Stalinism, before coming to this country, she was not the most emotionally stable of people. But through all that, her mind had stayed sharp as a razor, and it was a terrible shock to see her falling apart, not only physically but cognitively. Uncannily, she was still able to pick up on various things that were going on, albeit in a confused way. For example, she was convinced my father would have to go to court. In fact, what I hadn't told her was that a huge legal battle had flared up between me and my brother, over the management of my parents' affairs.

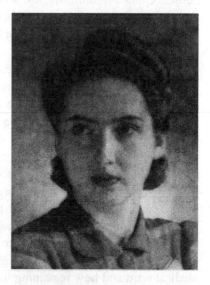

My brother and I disagreed about almost everything, while both being closely involved with my parents' care. In some ways, this was even harder than the immense amount of time and effort it took to set up care for them.

Maria's mother Ewa before the war

My brother's anxiety at their deterioration led him to search for someone he could find fault with – often the professionals involved, but more frequently myself. It seemed that nothing I could do was right in his eyes, and his constant accusations that our parents were getting worse because of my incompetence made the immense amount of work involved feel at times unbearable. It remains a great sadness that my parents' deteriorating health, and ultimately their deaths, did not bring us closer together, but drove us even further apart than we had ever been.

My father 'presented' very well to the world. A gentleman through and through, courteous and educated, he was still able to hold an interesting conversation about current affairs for a very short time. Minutes later he would forget whatever was being talked about and we would start again. It was exhausting. To my frustration, he would tell social workers and other professionals that he and my mother were managing perfectly well. He would have no recollection that my mother was by then actually using a wheelchair and couldn't go out by herself. He would tell them that she did all the shopping and housekeeping and that he managed the finances, when, of course, post would accumulate in piles that he was no longer able to deal with.

The hardest times were those of change. When my mother suddenly went into hospital, we had no care in place for my father, but it was obvious he couldn't manage on his own. My brother and I took turns to go and stay with him. When we couldn't be there, we'd phone to make sure he was taking his medication. A part-time carer was roped in to make meals and do the housekeeping for him. My life seemed to be falling apart. I'd come home from London and collapse with sheer exhaustion and then go back up again in a day or so. The only thing that kept me going was some strange kind of adrenalin.

There is such a steep learning curve, so much information to take in. Even simple things you hadn't realised, such as that constipation or a urinary infection, or not drinking enough water, affect a person's mental state so adversely. Hours and hours were spent trying to contact the various agencies to set up better care for my parents. Mostly the professionals were fantastic. The local Alzheimer's Concern listened and acknowledged what they were the first to name as the 'double whammy' of *both* my parents having dementia. There was a dementia advocate at the hospital who was brilliant, and helped to get things moving when the hospital bureaucracy ground to a halt. When my father was admitted to the same hospital (during my mother's long stay there) with a chest infection, he helped to arrange for my parents to see each other on the ward. He also understood the importance of getting my mother off the medical ward and how remaining in hospital was exacerbating her confusion.

Mysteriously, his post was later cut – a sad reflection on the continuing problem of under-resourcing.

Trying to get through to doctors on the phone will be a familiar nightmare to anyone who has been through this. They are so overworked you have to catch them in the maddeningly tiny window when they can speak to you. I had days of arranging my entire life around one precious phone call. Social services, despite my father's best attempts to tell them we had no need for their support, were also brilliant. In the end we set up a system of private full-time care, which my parents were lucky enough to be able to afford. My parents always said they didn't want to leave their home and be stuck with strangers and a whole load of 'old people'! We found Polish carers who lived in. This allowed my parents to stay in their own home, to eat familiar Polish food and not face the wrench of moving somewhere else. The carers were dedicated and motherly, and although at first my mother resented this – she wanted to be the one to look after my father – she did come round eventually and grew very fond of them. They in turn showed her affection and much understanding.

A social worker friend remarked that if all the Poles in Britain were to leave, the care system would collapse and social services would not be able to cope with the ensuing demands. When I visited my parents I took over, to give the carers as much respite as possible. Partly I felt guilty at not doing more; daughters – Polish daughters especially – tend to feel guilty most of the time. The carers worked all year round, including Christmas, and in their spare time they often took on extra work cleaning or looking after other people. My parents provided them with bed and board on top of their wages. What they saved, they sent home to the families they'd had to leave behind in order to provide for them by working abroad. This was particularly poignant when one of the carers lost her own mother during her time with us.

I also wanted to do things for my parents myself. Washing my mum's hair, giving my dad a back scrub, putting them to bed – there is something intimate and precious about caring for someone in a physical way. I feel privileged that I was able to do it sometimes, but that I didn't have to do it morning, noon and night. For years I'd argued with my parents about politics, about my sexuality. Their vulnerability put paid to that and all I could do, or wanted to do, was look after them. I was glad to find a big enough supply of love easily inside myself. At the same time, witnessing my parents' ever increasing dependence – eventually to the point of needing the most basic help in the toilet – made me cry as soon as I got home.

I was lucky, too, in that my partner Deborah had got to know my parents before the dementia really set in. At first my mother, especially, had been very frosty, while my father was more indifferent: neither of them liked the idea of my partner being another woman. Deborah decided not to take their attitude at face value and her persistent warmth and friendliness won them over. Her understanding and support made all the difference during the difficult times.

In some ways my father was luckier than my mother, because he had no idea how severe his memory loss had become. He would automatically deny anything was wrong, and remained convinced that he was coping. He seemed to be enjoying life with what could be called 'Zen beginner's mind'. He loved going swimming with my brother and his daughter, and was still able to swim gently up and down. One of the carers who came over from Poland had her children with her, and though he told them off for being too noisy, he liked seeing them. Instead of the two of them rattling around in their big old house there was a family atmosphere again. Each day started afresh with no recollection of what had happened even moments before. He could not remember the difficulties and differences in our family and this enabled him to have a sweet relationship with everyone. For the first time he became less of a traditional old-fashioned father. He no longer felt it was his parental duty to criticise, and became genuinely appreciative and grateful to anyone who showed him kindness and support.

I hoped against hope that when she came home from hospital, my mother would regain her mental abilities. She did become less agitated and was clearly happy to be home with my father, but she was never quite herself again. During the many mental assessments that my parents had to endure, a regular question was, 'Who is the prime minister of this country?' and I was heartened when my mother said the health professionals themselves should be quizzed as to who was the prime minister of Poland. There would be glimpses of that old self, flashes of humour and affection – which were heartbreaking for me, as they grew fewer over time.

She too was mellowed by the dementia in some ways. Or perhaps she withdrew into a more private world. Her memory still functioned better than my father's but she was more confused than him and suffered hallucinations from time to time. A shadow in the corner of the room might become a cat or even a dead body in her mind's eye. Others involved soldiers, priests and people from the past. She also experienced periods of lucidity when she realised how her mind was affected and found herself horrified at what was happening to her, as well as worrying about my father, which was something she had been doing throughout their relationship. They had met during the Warsaw resistance, when their lives were in constant danger, and her anxiety that something could happen to him never really left her.

There came times when she was sure he was going off to fight and he was helpless to reassure her. His own sense of time had diminished, and he would say stubbornly, 'I'll go if I need to,' or 'Well, I'm not going today,' which did nothing to dispel her certainty that the war was still going on.

I'd always worried my father might revert back to Russian, which he had spoken as a very young child, and that I wouldn't be able to understand him, but in fact it was my mother who became unintelligible to me. Whereas my father was able to converse quite normally, my mother struggled for words which would slip infuriatingly away from her and she would often say one thing when she meant another. If I was actually present it wasn't so bad, because I could point to things and try and guess what she meant. On the phone it became impossible to understand what she was saying. Sometimes I just asked her to say it again a different way and she'd get very frustrated with me and tell me how stupid I was – why did I not understand the most basic things? She also badgered my father, who had no recollection of her speech problems. After trying and trying to understand her, he would say irritably, 'What on earth are you talking about, woman?'

It took Deborah a while to realise how much guesswork was involved, as she would hear us talking in Polish and assume it was a normal conversation. Once during lunch when we were visiting, she asked me to translate. I had to tell her discreetly that I had no idea what my mum was talking about despite the fact that we'd been 'talking' for ages.

Frighteningly, I did occasionally get an inkling that what appeared total gibberish to me actually made sense. We'd go out for little 'walks', me push-ing the wheelchair and my father holding on to it, and my mother kept saying she wanted us to go and get the brothers. She was quite insistent about this. I racked my brains. No, she didn't mean my brother. She didn't mean any brother that I could come up with. One day we got it. She wanted us to go to Safeways and buy a bottle of wine: Ernest and Julio Gallo were the two brothers on the label of wine she remembered enjoying, and she wanted us to buy some more.

The hardest thing is witnessing the inevitability of a loved person's mental and physical deterioration. My father had done all the right things. At 70, having retired from being an engineer all his life, he enrolled at the local college to study computer programming. He also became chair of the Polish Underground Archive (which collects documents relating to the Polish resistance in World War II), successfully working on historical publications. It broke my heart when not only his short-term memory but even his long-term recollection finally went. I remember a conversation about the war when I realised he couldn't remember the Soviet army invading Poland in 1939. This was a fact so imprinted on his mind and the minds of his contemporaries. He himself had been rounded up by Soviet soldiers. I couldn't bear to see it had slipped away along with so much else.

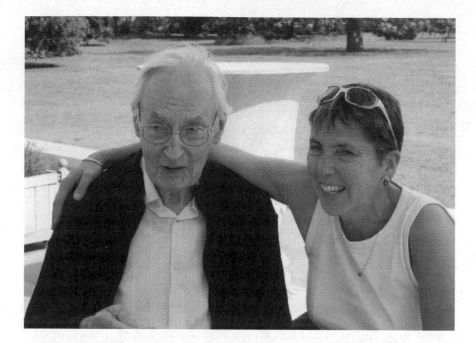

Maria with her father Leonard

All you can do is live in the moment. I knew that whatever we did, my father would certainly forget it in a very short space of time. But I believed it was worth doing and that the good moments would be lodged inside my parents' hearts, if not their minds. There were simple, companionable times, like sitting in my parents' garden with them. They would still 'read' the papers, and I would do some weeding and bring them cups of tea. Deborah and I took them on lots of outings. At Kew Gardens, we borrowed an extra wheelchair for my father to cover the immense distances. It took some persuading for him to use it as initially he insisted that Deborah sat in it and that he, ever the gentleman, would push *her*.

In Syon Park, we attended a 'meet the animals' session with a host of small children and their parents. The animal keepers brought out an amazing selection of creatures. My parents got to touch scorpions and centipedes, my mother proudly allowed an owl to sit on her wrist and my father had a python slither round his neck. Their delight equalled that of any of the children. Of course, when we showed them the photographs my dad remembered nothing, but it didn't matter. He'd been there. The image of my parents laughing was what I held on to.

There were embarrassing moments too. Towards the end of her life, my mother took to removing bits of food from the table and hiding them in her handbag. This, along with her false teeth shooting out with alarming speed, made me squirm a bit in restaurants and cafés. I remember two waiters turning away discreetly, their shoulders heaving with helpless laughter, as I scrabbled around on the floor looking for my mother's teeth. Deborah and I just laughed with them. My parents, not understanding the joke, caught the mood and laughed too, no doubt fortified by a little red wine. I was determined that my parents would not be hidden away at home.

My father was physically stronger than my mother and it was she who died before him. Her death was not unexpected. Given her age and frailty, I knew she would not last that year. Nevertheless, it was shattering. I also had to find a way to talk with my father about it, and this too was heartbreaking. She had died in hospital and he had not really known where she was. He was poorly himself and I had been worried he wouldn't be well enough to visit her. But with the help of the carers we had managed to get him into a cab and over to the hospital. My parents were so pleased to see each other. They held hands and cuddled like two little lovebirds. I don't know if either of them realised they were saying goodbye to each other.

On the morning of my mother's death, I had to tell my father. I knew that within an hour he would forget our conversation, but I also knew how it would affect him deep down. He was terribly shocked, as if he had been totally unprepared for it. After her death he would look for her in the house and ask the carers where she was. They were there with him seven days of the week and I think they made a decision to spare him as much as possible and allow him to think she might be coming back. When I came to visit him, I simply felt I couldn't lie to him. I couldn't bear to pretend my mother was alive. I didn't bring it up, but if he asked I told him the truth. Every conversation we had about her dying was like him hearing it for the first time and yet his reactions grew more subdued. I'm convinced that deep in his heart he knew, though his mind on another level could not retain it. In some ways the dementia cushioned him, as it had done through those last few years. He began to confuse the carers with my mother and regularly asked them to join him at bedtime. During my mother's funeral, my father had no idea what was going on, except when he noticed the hearse and announced that it must be somebody's funeral. A number of my parents' friends had come. We held the wake in the church social club and my father thoroughly enjoyed himself.

Sometimes I think he just assumed she was there, but if we went out he would suddenly notice she wasn't with us. I felt a light in him was fading – there is no other way to describe it. Once, looking out at the river, he said, 'Well, it's all over then.' Most of the time, however, he looked happy. Enjoying his walks, enjoying the attentions of the carers who shaved him, fed him, took him out, kissed him goodnight. On his last Christmas Eve, he happily buried his face in the bosoms of all the women around him. He wouldn't let them go and we couldn't start the special meal as he kept holding on to everyone. He died within a year of my mother.

I thought it would be a relief when they died, as they had both become so frail and ill by then. In some ways it is, when I hear friends going through the same battles to set up care, having to be permanently on call, waiting for the phone calls that say there has been another fall, an infection, another crisis. There were such long, draining hours spent in and out of hospital, spent on the phone, spent worrying. Watching your parents deteriorate is devastating, but I have friends who lost their parents much sooner than I did, and were devastated in a different way.

Now, when I walk along the seafront, I recall my parents' outings to Brighton, when their kind neighbour would drive them down. I've put up two commemorative plaques on a bench where my dad would sit with my mum in her wheelchair beside him, smiling not frowning. I remember his complete, delighted surprise on seeing the sea. They'd be eating ice cream and the wind would blow it everywhere. Not a day goes by without me missing them.

We Don't Know What is Going Through her Mind

Jennifer Davies

My parents had four children: two boys and two girls. I am the youngest and affectionately described as a 'mistake'. My parents lived for their children: we were simply the most important things in their lives.

Mom was an attractive woman and always very smart. She took great pride in her appearance. She kept a clean house and cooked good wholesome meals. She worked most of her life, as well as caring for her family and home, and retired from her job as a doctor's receptionist when she was 68.

Mom was a rather dominant character and very loving. She was a worrier, especially about her children. If we knew Mom was expecting us at a certain time and that we would be late, we tried somehow to contact her (no mobile phones in those days) because we knew she would simply assume that we had been killed. She would be climbing the walls, even after as short a time as fifteen minutes. And it was contagious. If we were waiting for my brother, and he was late, Mom would be so frantic with worry that Dad and I would start praying, too.

Mom hated staying in during the day, and once she had retired she went into town or one of the local shopping centres every day, come rain or shine. She was a great talker and always enjoyed a good chat whilst travelling on the bus. After these outings she would relay to us the conversations she had had. We always maintained that our family's business was known by strangers all over Birmingham because of Mom's 'chats' on the bus.

I find myself writing in the past tense, although Mom is still living. I suppose I do so because of Mom's condition now and how different she is. But although very different, mentally and physically, from what I describe above, she is still Mom. This is simply another phase of her life. However, I do miss

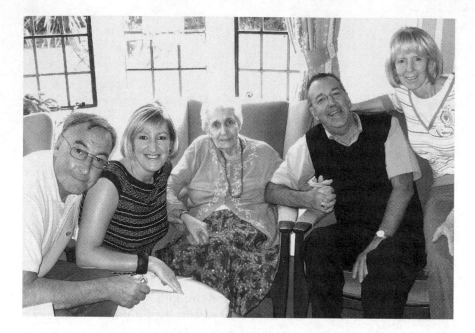

Patricia Scully with her children (L to R) John, Jennifer, Mick and Sheila

her and it does tend to feel a little like bereavement. She loved the Carpenters and often when we went out in the car I would put on their CD and we would sing along. Now whenever a Carpenters' song comes on the radio I feel like crying. I often used to bump into Mom in Marks and Spencer when I popped out in my lunchtime to buy a sandwich. She was always so happy to see me, even for that brief time. On several occasions I have felt near to tears in M&S, thinking that I will never meet her in there again.

The terrible dementia from which Mom suffers began about eight years ago.

One day she had a fall whilst out shopping. There was a hole in the pavement outside the chemist shop. It was a dark, rainy day, and down she went. She broke her hip and had to have an operation. I suppose it was during her time in hospital that we first noticed how she was beginning to forget words – simple, obvious words like 'cup'. I recall one evening when we were all visiting together and Mom was trying to remember the name of a particular country. You know what it's like when a word is on the tip on your tongue but you just can't grasp it, and we knew it was driving her mad. So we began to offer suggestions. In the end we got it: Zimbabwe! I remember saying I was glad we hadn't started to list countries alphabetically, as we would have been there until midnight, and everybody laughed.

Mom and Dad were Catholics, Dad especially devout, and we were brought up in the faith. I can recall going to Mass with her and hearing her faltering over the prayers. This was unusual because Mom had a tendency to pray loudly and quickly. She always finished the 'Our Father' before the rest of the congregation were halfway through. As a child I found this desperately embarrassing and would send her evil looks throughout Mass – very holy!

Life seemed to carry on as normal, but Mom began to deteriorate. She became obsessed with certain things. It started with the wrinkles on her face. She would have no other topic of conversation. However hard we tried to convince her that her wrinkles were no worse than those of anyone else her age, that it was normal and they weren't that bad anyway, she couldn't accept it or understand why it had happened to her. Then, after some months, she moved on to her breasts. She was perplexed as to why they were so large and hung down. She took to getting her breasts out in public to illustrate to others what she was talking about. We had visions of her being arrested and the headline reading, 'Pensioner jailed for exposing herself in public'. But, on the whole, people were very kind.

Then she became very upset by the television. When it was on, she was under the illusion that those on screen were addressing her directly and she wouldn't be rude and turn away. On many occasions when I called in I was unable to have a conversation with Mom because Richard and Judy were talking to her! And when the television was switched off she was alarmed at her reflection and thought it was another person. We had to cover up the television with a tea towel.

While all this was happening, Dad passed away. Mom now lived alone in a warden-controlled flat. Luckily, the warden was a nice woman who was fond of Mom and was happy for her to live there as long as was possible. But she was worried when Mom continued to go out each day, catching the bus to the local shopping centre or into Birmingham city centre. She started to express some concern about Mom getting lost or in difficulty. And she was right because it wasn't long before Mom was brought home by the police, having been found in a rather confused state outside the chemist's.

During this time, Mom had a lot of support from her family, even though we were all working full-time. Mom was lucky that she had four children, and we were lucky to have each other. We all helped Mom and communicated with each other on a more or less daily basis, especially my sister and me. We are very close, and all lived quite near. However, it was becoming clear that Mom needed more help if she was to continue living in her flat. We arranged for someone to go in each morning to help, and we took it in turns to call in after work to ensure that she had something to eat. She has always loved being surrounded by her children and was happy that we always seemed to be there.

Once I was chatting about my husband, and Mom suddenly asked me who I was talking about:

'Rob, Mom.'

'Who's Rob?'

'My husband!'

'Your husband!' Mom exclaimed with an astonished look on her face. 'I didn't know you had got married. Well, fancy not telling me you had got married.'

'Mom, love, I got married seven years ago. You were there. Look, here's our wedding photograph. You saw Rob last week!' Mom looked sheepish but we both began to laugh.

And then Mom had a fall and broke her leg. That marked the end of Mom's independent life.

She was admitted to hospital, and it was a time of anguish for us all. Mom was simply unable to understand what had happened to her and why she was there. Leaving her each evening was like leaving a small, frightened child. It affected us all and, even now, it is disturbing to think back to it. We felt so powerless. When we were at work, thoughts of Mom filled our minds. It was hard to concentrate and everything else seemed unimportant. Mom was in hospital for about four weeks, and the care was appalling. She was a difficult patient because of her dementia and the nursing staff simply didn't seem to know how to deal with her. After a few weeks Mom was transferred to a different hospital. She was there for ten weeks and the nursing staff were relatively kind and patient, even though from time to time Mom threw terrible tantrums if they asked her to do anything she didn't want to, especially physiotherapy. If it hurt, Mom simply would not do it.

We were all well aware that Mom would never return to her flat and we had to start the depressing task of finding residential accommodation for her. We were lucky to find a really nice home, which she moved into when she left hospital.

At first, Mom was not only confused, but also appeared timid, too. She stopped eating and lost a lot of weight. I recall on one occasion Mom wasn't very well and had been sick. They moved her to her room to give her some privacy and made her comfortable. When we arrived to see her she was warm and comfortable, but she thought she had done something wrong and was being punished by being moved away from the others and put in her room on her own. We were distraught to see Mom like this.

Now, after two years, Mom is thriving and will celebrate her eighty-sixth birthday this year. In a way she has become institutionalised and is used to her surroundings. We are too. We know the staff well and they are used to us. We go to see Mom very regularly. She remains alert and recognises us all and is always pleased to see us, although she can't say our names. She is still a talker, but unfortunately we can't understand what she is saying. From time to time a lucid sentence comes out and we get the idea. But the love is there in her eyes and smile. She will always raise her face for a kiss, run her fingers through our hair, hold our hands, comment – in her own way – on what we are wearing. So I suppose, after so much trauma, it is more peaceful now.

But no one wants to see their parents end up in a nursing home in this condition. For the first few months I used to wake at two or three in the morning and lie there for hours worrying and grieving about Mom. I would imagine her waking in the night and being frightened. Would the staff be kind to her? I wanted to install secret cameras to check she was being cared for properly.

Dementia is such a dreadful disease, rendering the sufferer childlike. But a baby can cry when hungry or thirsty, Mom can't. She has to remain hungry and thirsty until she is fed and watered. She is incontinent, which still greatly upsets her. We don't know what is going through her mind. What if it is fear and we can't reassure her? What if she is in pain and can't make anyone understand? Babies are cute and appealing. Elderly people often aren't. Mom can't get enjoyment from reading, watching the television, listening to music. She doesn't enjoy her food, which has to be liquidised; she can't enjoy a sherry before lunch, appreciate a nice bunch of flowers or have a really good chat. That is always at the back of my mind, and often jumps to the forefront: while I have been having a busy, enjoyable day, Mom has been sitting in her armchair all the time. But maybe my worries are unfounded. Maybe the dementia has taken away Mom's cravings for these things I mention. We just don't know.

I understand that some who suffer with dementia become aggressive or violent, that they can't remember their family at all and become almost comatose. Thankfully this hasn't happened to Mom – or at least, not yet! She seems to have remained the same for the last couple of years, getting no worse. I hope so much that this continues to be the case.

3

The Departing Light

Jim Swift

On 11 April 2002 I learned that my wife, Jan, had dementia. She was 58 years old.

The first indication of something odd had come when we went on holiday to Italy in 1996. One night we went out for a meal, and Jan suddenly asked me where we had been the previous day. We had in fact visited Venice, and had enjoyed a memorable day out. Jan had bought me a tie on the Rialto Bridge. I looked at Jan and saw the utter fear in her eyes as she struggled to remember this fantastic day. I told her where we had been and her face cleared as the memories came back to her. I think even at this early stage I knew that the omens were bad: I lay awake most of the night thinking of what this might mean.

As the years passed, the incident went to the back of my mind. Jan and I were both teachers by profession and had often worked together over the course of our careers. By 2000, Jan was working as a supply teacher in various schools in Manchester, Salford and Bolton. She was still functioning normally on one level, but it was obvious that something was wrong. She could get confused as to which supply agency she was working for, and she would sometimes double-book a day at two schools. She was also forgetting to pay some bills and was buying food that we had already got, so that we could end up with a dozen tins of tuna!

The doctor eventually referred her to the psychiatric department of the local hospital, where they concluded that she was suffering from depression and dissatisfaction with supply teaching. It took several more visits before a brain scan was performed. This showed a perfectly normal brain. Throughout all the hospital visits I had been keeping my thoughts to myself, but now that Jan had been given the all-clear, I told her what my fears had been. Jan replied that she was glad I hadn't told her as she wouldn't have wanted to know.

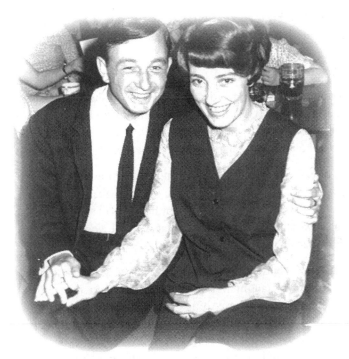

Jim and Jan on their honeymoon, 1969

Despite this verdict, Jan's abilities continued to decline. She was sent for a deeper scan, and this time the results indicated Alzheimer's. After the initial devastation, and after informing family and friends, I quickly decided that I would never tell Jan about her condition as she had made her wishes perfectly clear on this matter. This was going to be difficult, as we had always shared everything throughout our marriage. It would mean lying 'big time' to the person I loved most in the world. However, I came to the conclusion that this was for the best, as if she knew the truth, then every time she forgot something or did something silly she would imagine it was just one more step on the road to oblivion.

Jan was put under the care of a consultant and received regular home visits where her memory and abilities were tested. She was also prescribed Aricept, which for a while actually improved her scores on the tests.

In the summer of 2004, we visited Eastbourne for the annual air display. I left Jan sitting on a bench on the promenade whilst I went for some sandwiches. When I returned, Jan had wandered off into the large crowd that had gathered. With the help of a policeman I got an announcement put over the tannoy system but I spotted Jan before the announcement could produce any results. The fear that gripped me was not a feeling I want to experience again.

That year, I wrote:

Jan is still the same loving and caring person that she always was. Her personality has not changed, but it is heartbreaking to see her struggle to remember the names of everyday objects. She cannot deal with money, tell the time, work any household appliances or write her name. I cannot leave her alone.

As the disease does not follow a set pattern, and the symptoms people exhibit vary, you don't know what to expect, which makes looking into the future even more scary. If Jan could remain at her present level, then, hard as this is to bear, it would be wonderful. My fear is that I won't be able to cope when the disease really takes hold.

Since then, Jan's abilities have declined markedly. Jan was a head teacher in two schools, and taught hundreds of children to read, write and compute. Now, she cannot do these things herself. At the present time she cannot even dress herself. Left to her own devices she would put her clothes on over her pyjamas. She would put one cardigan on over another, one pair of trousers over another. She would forget to wipe herself after visiting the toilet if not supervised. Twice I have loaded up her toothbrush with toothpaste, only to see her try to wet it with water in the toilet. She sometimes looks at me and asks me, 'Where's Jim?' She has a fascination with our remote control devices and will take them around with her. Objects disappear, only to be found in some peculiar location. She follows me everywhere and tries to help. Jan cannot recognise an object even if I point to it and give its colour. She is increasingly querulous and aggressive when I help her to dress or undress. A lot of the time her conversation does not make much sense.

Recently, at the day centre that Jan attends twice a week, a member of staff told me that she spent a lot of her time talking to another client, a man of roughly the same age, but that her conversation was 'mostly gibberish'. I had never categorised Jan's speech with this word, and the word itself shocked and upset me more than some of the more outlandish things that Jan does. But every day now there is hurt. It is difficult not to cry when your wife tells you that you are stupid, rubbish, a mess and that you do nothing. It is devastating to see every last vestige of humanity slowly stripped away from this caring, confident and intelligent woman.

Early on I adopted the mantra 'DIM – Does it really matter?' Does it really matter if Jan carries the remotes around? But often this is easier to say than achieve. When the television picture disappears for the umpteenth time that day or when her engagement ring gets lost again, things can get to you.

I cannot bear the thought of Jan having to enter a home. It would feel like I had betrayed and abandoned her, and so I have spent all our savings on the construction of a downstairs bedroom and walk-in shower. I don't know if I will be strong enough to deal with what still lies ahead, but I owe it to Jan to try. Silly as it sounds, at one time I did not think that I could even put her earrings into her pierced ears, but you learn to cope because you have to.

I would not even have been able to get this far without the support of our Admiral nurse. Her advice, expertise, professionalism, care and compassion have guided me and given me the strength to get so far. This is a service which should be expanded to cover the whole country and should be a priority of the government's carers' strategy.

It is hard now to remember what the original Jan was like, except when we watch home videos, but I can't bear to watch for long as the difference between Jan then and now is too painful to observe for long.

I am corresponding by email with a man whose wife also has Alzheimer's and I find this long-range sharing of experience really cathartic. Although family and friends tell me to feel free to talk to them about Jan, I am reluctant to do so as I feel they must be bored to death listening to my outpourings.

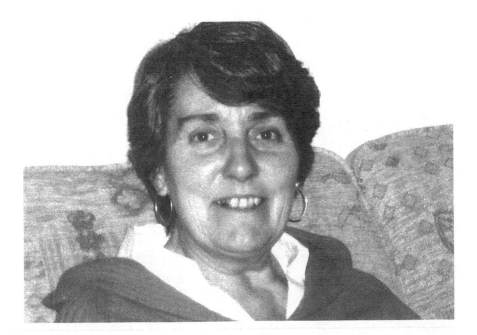

Jan, 2007

My elder daughter finds it especially difficult to hear how her mum has deteriorated and so I find myself keeping my thoughts to myself. My younger daughter lives in Kent and so is protected by distance from most of the pain.

At the funeral of Ronald Reagan, who also suffered from Alzheimer's, his wife Nancy called it 'the departing light', and this was how I came to choose this title for my chapter. It is also the way I think of Jan. She lit up the lives of hundreds of children during her teaching career. She was the best nursery and infant teacher I ever met, and when her light is finally extinguished, then the world will be a lesser place.

Jan is still just about in the real world. She still has the same warm personality, with a love especially of children. I treasure every moment, but even after six years, I wake up devastated by this illness that has blighted our lives. If there is one good thing to cling to, it is that I have been able to say and do things that I might not have said or done if Jan had died suddenly.

Since I received the news, I have tried my best to provide whatever Jan has requested. In the words of the song by Sting, 'I swear in the days still left, we will walk in fields of gold.' I have tried to make every day golden.

Walking on Thin Ice

Rachael Dixey

I'm scared that if I go away for a fortnight, Irene will have forgotten me when I return. Just now when I see her, she recognises me and either stops in amazement from her incessant walking up and down, and we hug, or she grabs my hand joyfully, kisses it, and says, 'Come on!' and charges off with me in tow, down the corridor. Then we sit, and she always says something like, 'Oh, I do love you!' or, 'You are the one – I just want to be with you.' This is all I have left – and if it went too, I would be desolate. She also enjoys seeing me and I feel bad thinking she'll miss me for two weeks. *But* I need a break – I am tired, catching every cold going and I want to stop so much, to sit by a warm blue sea and just watch the waves...

Caring for a loved one who has dementia means nothing is ever quite right – you know you need a break but you also feel you need to be there, caring. If you want company and go out, you wonder what you're doing there, and want to get away from everyone. If you're on your own, you wish you had company. Nothing is right, simply because nothing *is* right. The person you love is still there – but not there.

Irene lives in her own world, inaccessible to me, but she can still come out of that world so that we can be together – for about an hour, or less, and then she needs to retreat to her world. This means walking up and down the corridors, talking to herself in words no one else can understand, laughing often and sometimes singing. And the world of the dementia ward is often a place where I feel more comfortable myself, being with the care staff and the other patients. In the 'real', outside world, it feels as if people can only understand to a certain extent, and then they feel uncomfortable.

When I first met Irene, we knew we would spend our lives together, and we have done, very happily. Even after more than twenty years, my heart and eyes would light up whenever I saw her. They still do, but now there are other, more complex feelings there too. To know that we matter profoundly to another person gives meaning to our lives, and dementia robs us of certainty: do I still matter profoundly to Irene or does she kiss everyone's hand? I believe I still matter profoundly to her, and that anyone with dementia has an emotional memory which remains after other types of memory have gone. And *her* eyes light up still, for the moment.

So what has been our story so far? How did we get to this point, where the love of my life is in her world and the love of hers is here, in our home, alone? Where to start is blurry, because for so long the symptoms didn't seem that different from what many fifty-somethings are going through – the jokes about going upstairs and forgetting what you've gone for. But dementia isn't just about memory: it's about your ability to think, about cognition. It became clearer that Irene's problems were not just to do with being disorganised, or being hard of hearing or losing confidence. Her driving skills went. She was an experienced teacher of literature, but she literally began to lose the plot – not only could she not remember a story, she couldn't *understand* it. We went to see the film *Iris*,[1] and in the way that long-term couples have, we left the cinema without saying a word, but with a shared understanding that we knew what we were going to face too.

She saw a specialist in November 2003 for tests which confirmed cause for concern; in April 2004 the consultant suggested it was Alzheimer's. Irene

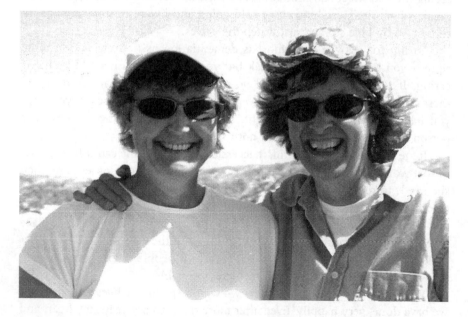

Rachael (left) and Irene in Blackpool, 2006

was 56. I can remember clearly sitting there, thinking, 'This is the nightmare coming true.' Irene immediately dismissed the verdict and wanted to move on with her life. This set the tone, and we *never* used the 'A' word again. Losing your partner is one thing, but it's doubly hard never discussing this with the one in whom you normally confide everything.

Needing help, I saw my GP in February 2005, still trying to pretend that there might be nothing 'really' wrong. She said that in three or four years' time, Irene would be in residential care. I was stunned, tried to continue my journey into work, but instead, ended up crying on the sofa of friends. For this blunt confirmation, I was grateful. Later that year, being outside 'the system' and needing help, I referred myself to the clinical psychologist in the Younger People with Dementia team, who involved the community psychiatric nurse (CPN), who agreed to see Irene at home. By then, Irene was in a state where it was easy to explain the presence of professionals simply by saying that they would help. Irene no longer had the capacity to really ask questions, had lost insight. So started a long period with the CPN, who has been terrific, and the psychiatrist, also a lovely woman, coming out about once a month and seeing us at home.

That sets out the facts and dates. The emotional turmoil is much more difficult to describe, as are the practical ways in which we coped. I work four days a week in a demanding job. Being seven years younger than Irene, I was nowhere near retirement age and anyway did not consider giving up my job – financially not possible, but also I knew it would do neither of us any good to be together all the time. Through 2006, Irene increasingly couldn't cope on her own and, by September, we needed a rota of paid helpers and friends so that she wasn't ever alone for more than half an hour – psychologically, she needed company. We'd already relied on friends and family for chunks of the day and, in between, she would ring me persistently at work, sometimes in great distress. This was awful, as I could do nothing from that distance. In March 2007 I also enlisted a couple of agencies that give carers time off, which enabled me to have an evening off each week. Otherwise, I relied on finding amazingly patient, kind people who could cope with the way Irene's sweet nature and hilarity would suddenly swing into fury and frustration. Eventually, after a lengthy process, we got direct payments to help with the costs. Looking back, I realise the strain of organising all this. My life over the last few years has become totally bound up with coping with Irene's illness, having slipped day by day from being primarily a 'partner' to being principally a 'carer'.

I can't really encapsulate all the things that happened during these years. There were many crises and many heartbreaks. A few stand out. Once we were sitting on our patio in the sunshine. Irene was aware that she was slipping; she was upset. She pleaded, 'I don't know who I am any more. Please help me.' I'm sobbing now as I remember this, as I couldn't at the time. I was needed then, to hug her, hold her, try to help her to keep the threads together. But it was perhaps the saddest day of my life. This strong, funny, intelligent woman, losing who she was.

Even after all these years, I *still* find it hard to believe that Alzheimer's has happened to *us*, as if we were sent the wrong script. *We* were the couple destined to spend 60 years together, to fade into the sunset... I felt that we were like two trees, strong individuals on the surface, but with our roots totally intertwined underneath, me inconceivable without her.

Another time, not so long ago, we set off from our home in Yorkshire for the Lake District – always a special place for us. Irene was brought up there and it was the location of many happy times for us. Irene forced me to stop seven times, insisting we were going the wrong way. She would try to get out of the car, banging her fists; once stopped, she would storm off down the busy highway. I would cajole her back in, set off, try again, double back. We came home twice, and once drove for miles in what I knew was the wrong direction, but it kept her happy. A kind of madness takes over – you do anything to keep the peace, hold your breath, hope for the crazy minutes to pass into something more recognisable. Symbolic that we could no longer get to the place which was so special for us.

The abrupt change when Irene went into hospital, here one day and not the next, was profoundly shocking. It was 29 August 2007, the day Irene left our home, stopped living with me – a day I will always remember; a kind of ending, one of many, but this one overwhelmingly brutal. I wrote the following piece at the time, in an attempt to come to terms with it:

> The decision which we all know looms on some horizon at some hazy future date has been made, almost by stealth. Irene has been admitted and it looks like she might never come home again. The stealth was not intentional. A crisis stretching into weeks rather than the odd day of furious behaviour, upset and exhaustion, fuelled by Irene's paranoia ('I WANT YOU TO CALL THE POLICE!') led to the scheduled visit from our psychiatrist resulting in a recommendation that Irene should go into hospital, to 'get her medication sorted out'. Irene had packed a bag before the doctor had even left the house. She clearly wanted to be off, out of the house where I was someone malign and 'out to get her' and where she alternately shouted, 'THIS IS NOT MY HOUSE!' or 'THIS IS MY HOUSE – GET OUT!' and from which she had locked me out the week before.
>
> Still in some sort of denial, and scared of the consequences of Irene leaving home for any length of time (and so forgetting it forever), I prevaricated

and could only see the short periods of calm as evidence that Irene really 'wasn't too bad'. I wasn't seeing the fear, confusion and deterioration that so plainly showed that Irene had entered another new phase. I was incapable of making a decision. Our CPN was due to call that afternoon and I decided that I would do whatever she recommended. To her it was clear – Irene needed to be in hospital.

Just before we left the house, Irene and I were alone in the living room, and *she* comforted me, saying, 'It's okay, Rach, it won't be for long and we'll always have each other.' I was astounded: just seconds before she didn't seem to even know who I was.

My sister came to help, sitting in the back seat of the car with Irene as I drove. I know it's not safe to drive with blinding tears, and my poor sister had either me to worry about or Irene, who changed from wanting to be journeying to safety to being extremely agitated and trying to get out of the car. Leaving her at the hospital was excruciating and Irene herself kept saying to the admissions doctor, 'Well, thank you very much but we have to be going now,' and picking up her little bag and making for the door.

Next morning, Irene was very distressed and kept repeating, 'I HAVE DONE NOTHING WRONG!' believing that she had been sent away to be punished. The consultant's quick assessment was that Irene was not out of place on an acute ward. He stunned me by saying that getting the medication right would take two or three months, not two or three weeks. I asked him to give me things straight, and he said it was unlikely that Irene could go home after this, ever. There – the decision about when Irene should go into care, which had felt like a massive hurdle in the future, was suddenly made and was behind us. And this is where this disease is so hard – there's uncertainty and shocks every step of the way.

This was the last day of August. Two weeks previously, we had been cycling in Holland, albeit with Irene on the wrong side of the road. Two weeks before that we had been canoeing on the river Wharfe (we are experienced canoeists, I hasten to add!), in our new inflatable canoe and Irene had loved it, the peace and quiet of a backwater, floating along, watching swans preening in the evening summer light.

I asked the consultant how it was possible to deteriorate this quickly. He said something really useful: that it's like walking on thin ice and the ice is getting thinner and thinner but you don't especially notice – until suddenly you fall through, and your world is suddenly so, so different. He said that because Irene had a high IQ and that we had such a good system of care at home, the cracks had been harder to see.

I spent a whole week bending everyone's ear about whether we had made the right decision to admit Irene; it was blindingly obvious to everyone except me. I thought we could surely have still managed at home, that she didn't really need to be with all these other ill folk, far from home. I then had another week of feelings of relief, some of the stress lifting, of being extraordinarily tired, and of looking back and realising that I had seen the cracks opening up in the ice, and of course we had had some terrible times of crisis behaviour that somehow I had just managed, because your sense of what's 'normal' and what's a 'crisis' becomes completely distorted when you live with someone with Alzheimer's. I had held my breath, carried on doing the things which Irene herself wanted to do, tried to keep a quality of life, with friends and relatives sometimes being amazed at what we did still manage to achieve. And of course, you just do it, if you love someone.

Three weeks have passed. Irene is different daily. One day she put her arms round me in the corridor and said, 'I love you.' She asked how long she would have to be there, and said, 'We have a lovely home.' Another day she wasn't even aware of me. She has deteriorated further as the inevitable institutionalisation creeps in and she leaves behind the one-to-one care at home. Three weeks, and I'm beginning to allow myself to grieve for my partner in a way that I couldn't while she was still at home – still here but not the person she was, a partner lost but present.

If we knew what was round the corner in life – and if we knew that that future contained Alzheimer's – would we despair? Probably, so it's just as well that we don't know. I was lamenting to my sister-in-law, grieving for our future together, that I wanted another 30 years of retirement together rather than just our 30 years of life together so far, and she said, 'Well, you don't know that would have happened anyway – Irene might have died from something else, or canoed off into the sunset with someone else.' (Unlikely, but you never know.) I found this surprisingly cheering. What I do know is that even if I had known that we were to be sent the script with Alzheimer's in the story line instead of the script that I'd hoped for, I would still have chosen to spend my life with Irene, the best partner anyone could ever have wished for.[2]

This new phase, on my own, is harder than I'd expected. The speed of Irene's decline is difficult to take in; rather than the 'three or fours years' of the GP's prediction, we had two and a half. I miss Irene with all my heart, and it's tougher than I can say visiting her, though I need to go, and do almost every day. She moved from the acute ward to a community psychiatric unit after two months, and was much happier. The drug regime seems to be working and on the whole she is content. My worry doesn't stop, and I am trying to get her a permanent placement. There are several pieces of the jigsaw that need to happen – assessments, the finance – and I will be relieved once all this has happened. Recently she has been aggressive with the staff who have to dress her and help her with the toilet. You never know what will happen next, and no one can tell you. You live in a constant state of confusion, of feelings and emotions, of not knowing whether to plan this and that, or just let others take over, of never knowing what you will find the next time you see your loved one, and of having no means of preparing for it all.

It is heart-rending but wonderful to see the Irene of old, her character and humour still there in flashes, still the loving, affectionate and headstrong person she always was. She makes the staff smile. She and I are often in fits of giggles; often she makes me cry. This inner core that is left suggests she must have been a happy child.

At the moment I'm still caught up in the 'now', and it's too painful to look back on the happier times, our civil partnership day, and earlier, our twenty-fifth anniversary, our house filled with flowers and friends; all the walking and sailing we did, all the togetherness. I have put a photo of Irene in every room in the house, and am gearing myself for this strange twilight, where Irene is alive but increasingly moving away. I have to sort out my life as a singleton, yet still I have a partner. I have to steady myself for the real ending, because Alzheimer's shortens the sufferer's life, and that is where the final grieving will begin. But I know that I have enough love left from Irene to warm me through the rest of my life.

Notes

[1] The film about the novelist Iris Murdoch, showing how she succumbed to Alzheimer's disease.

[2] Thanks to Alzheimer's Society for permission to reproduce this text, which first appeared anonymously in Alzheimer's Society LGBT carers' group newsletter, July 2008.

5

The Most Difficult Decision of my Life

Debbie Jackson

When my husband and I arrived in England, accompanied by our three children, we were in our late thirties. It was the very first time we had been outside South Africa, the country of our birth. This was the 1960s, and South Africa was pretty much a police state under the rule of a determined and ruthless apartheid government.

My husband was a lawyer and had successfully run his own law practice in Cape Town for fifteen years; I was a social worker, dealing with problems of poverty and ill-health. We had both been active in the anti-apartheid struggle. B had been one of the few lawyers prepared to act in the courts in defence of people accused of offences regarded as 'political'. He also spoke out boldly in committees and, when the need arose, on public platforms, against the ever-increasing unjust and oppressive measures the government was introducing.

Eventually, and inevitably, like many other anti-apartheid activists, he was served with a 'banning order'. This meant he was prohibited from attending any gathering – a dangerously vague term, leaving our friends and relations afraid even to visit the house in case he was arrested. Further clauses prevented him from being quoted in any publication, being present on educational premises (which of course affected our children), entering docks or airports, and communicating with other banned persons (I remember clandestine meetings at a carpet shop near his law office). Furthermore, he had to report to the police every Monday – a great nuisance, particularly on holiday Mondays, when it was easy to forget! A breach of any of these conditions could incur arrest and imprisonment.

B had always shown courage and optimism – and also plenty of humour – in the face of any challenges life presented. And when we came to England, he tackled the hurdle of re-qualifying in his profession and starting to practise law here in the same spirit. We steadily adapted and built up a new life here in London.

He relished a good argument, and with his clear and incisive mind he would quickly get to the heart of any discussion or debate. His friends remember that he was enormous fun, with a very individual way of expressing his opinions. They mention too his deep-seated sense of loyalty, his respect and love for justice, his lack of pomposity and the way he upheld his principles without wavering. Friends and clients still remember, too, his wise advice – sensible, measured, down-to-earth and tempered by a wry sense of humour.

How sad to be writing all this, of necessity, in the past tense.

For so much of it is lost to us, now that he is in the advanced stages of dementia. The twinkle in the eyes is still sometimes discernible (and these are precious moments!) but the powers of communication are now so depleted that we can have little knowledge of what he might be thinking, feeling, or wishing to convey. But I must add that some major aspects of his personality have noticeably remained unaffected – for instance, his enjoyment of company has not been quite extinguished. His emotional response to the music he always loved is also still manifest.

Of course, these changes have not taken place all at once.

By the 1990s, we were in our sixties, approaching the time when we could hope to enjoy our retirement years together after both working hard throughout our marriage. Little had we dreamed what overwhelming heartaches awaited us. Over the next few years my dear B showed increasing signs of the vascular dementia he was eventually diagnosed with in 1996, which was to devastate the comfort and companionship of our happy married life together, and which led to a drastic shift in our roles, responsibilities and relationships.

In the early stages, his developing dementia showed itself only sporadically (so that those visitors who came infrequently sometimes doubted why I was worried, as there seemed to be nothing wrong), and took the form of diminished self-confidence and enthusiasm, less keenness to participate, less ability to find his own way, inability to make decisions, inability to learn anything new (such as how to operate the switches on any new appliance), and of course the perpetually repeated questions which resulted from loss of short-term memory. I remember in particular how he became less and less willing to answer the phone, if he knew he was going to be asked by a friend for legal advice (he would formerly have been so spontaneous in his help, even though he was now officially retired) and would ask me to make some excuse because he obviously could not face the conversation.

My feelings at this stage were of unease, uncertainty, a sense of impending loss, a constant and generalised anxiety, and – yes – sometimes uncontrollable irritation, particularly at the repetitive questions. (Naturally, this irritation led to the inevitable sense of guilt felt by all carers in this situation.)

When the formal diagnosis of vascular dementia was made, my feelings were of devastation and catastrophe. I was overcome with a great fear of the future, as well as deep sorrow and sympathy for my husband in what seemed a kind of death sentence – and who knew how long the loss and suffering would continue? I also felt a desperate need to protect him from experiencing the same feeling of despair that was overwhelming me. And this marked my attitude, also, to the task of telling our adult children. They were aware, of course, that something was very wrong, but the diagnosis when it came was such a horribly definite blow, holding out so little hope over the long term, that the whole family were naturally terribly upset. I have had wonderful and unstinting support from them throughout, and they see their father as often as they can – and often speak to him on the phone too, as he clearly enjoys hearing their voices.

In many ways, those early days when he still had some degree of insight into his condition, and needed reassurance, were the hardest. I recall an awful moment (repeated at intervals) when he said in obvious distress: 'What's happening to me? Am I going mad?' I did what I could to explain matters to him in a way that he could comprehend, but my heart was breaking. And my own feelings of anxiety seemed to reinforce his anxieties, try as I might not to show them. Thus our tension was at a high level.

Our GP was a great source of help, but we were all too soon in need of further help from the local authority social services who provided carers for personal care, as he became less able to do things for himself. Crossroads proved a wonderful provider of a 'sitting service' to keep B company while I got out of the flat for a couple of hours on a regular basis for household shopping, or just to be on my own or with a friend. The Admiral nurse who gave me unstinting support was a godsend, and then there were the occupational therapists and even a community psychiatric nurse, who all on occasion contributed much-appreciated input.

I could not have done without this type of help. But there is no denying that I had to adjust to a totally different way of life, with much less privacy in the home, and a great deal of responsibility as a coordinator of multiple services, which obviously did not always proceed smoothly. I also found myself sometimes feeling resentful that I had lost my independence in running my own home.

Perhaps the most important and lasting contribution to our wellbeing throughout this 'journey' has been that of Jewish Care, a London-based welfare organisation which has provided us with so much help. For a while, B would attend one day a week at one of their excellent day care centres, specifically geared to the needs of people with dementia. This gave him pleasant activities and company, while I was able to spend several hours at a time just doing whatever I liked or needed, as long as I was there to pick him up at the end of the day.

As a carer, I was catered for by Jewish Care in an invaluable support group meeting once a month. This group still continues, and gives carers who wish to attend the support of mutual understanding, and enables us to express our feelings and reactions to sometimes traumatic events, in a safe and confidential setting.

One of the seemingly inevitable results of the impact of dementia on the carer (particularly in the case of spouses) is the sense of isolation as one's old social life becomes impossible. Friends sometimes try to keep in touch but often without success, as many people just 'can't handle it' when confronted with the difficulties of communication with their old friend who has developed this daunting condition. A good carers' support group goes a long way towards counteracting the sadness and loneliness this brings.

By 1999, things had become a lot harder to deal with, as B was needing much more help. In particular his mobility had suffered, and he now became quite unable to go downstairs from our flat, which meant we could no longer leave the building together. He was now virtually a prisoner in his own home – which made me a partial prisoner too! Till then we had gone for daily walks in the neighbourhood together; and I worried as to what would happen if there was a fire or other emergency. At this point I began to suffer waves of despair.

Somewhat reluctantly, I was persuaded to arrange for a couple of spells of respite care for him (two weeks at a time) at a local Jewish Care home, to enable me to take much-needed breaks. They did help me to recharge my batteries, and I had to agree it was necessary. But they were worrying times, knowing he was in unfamiliar surroundings and without his being able to understand where or why.

Eventually, in 2000, the problems of his mobility, anxiety, incontinence and now occasional aggression (always followed swiftly by remorse and reconciliation) became really bad, and I had to admit I was no longer coping well. He now needed much more personal care and I in turn developed severe sciatica and became depressed and distraught.

Eventually our GP called in a psychogeriatrician, who visited and assessed B, and recommended he enter a care home on a long-term basis, as soon as possible. To accept this was the most difficult decision of my life. Naturally I discussed it with the family, and it was heartbreaking for us all, but was obviously inevitable. A couple of months later, a vacancy came up at the Jewish

Care home I had applied for. B was admitted there in December 2000, and astonishingly is still there today.

I will never forget the day we took him to the home. Because of his difficulty negotiating our stairs, I had arranged for a private ambulance, and we were accompanied by a favourite carer (a confident young Nigerian man, a part-time law student) whom B and I had taught the old South African song 'Sarie Marais'. The bemused and amused paramedics were treated to repeated choruses of 'Sarie Marais' on the journey. It did keep his spirits up – and concealed my struggle not to cry!

The management of the care home had a good welcome ready, showing us up to his room, where we found a lovely bowl of fresh fruit waiting on the dressing table. A nurse and a key worker already allocated to B were on hand, helping to unpack his case and settle him in. When, with breaking heart, I could be prised away, the social worker drove me home: home to the flat I would be living in alone.

Apart from the two months when B had of necessity preceded me and the children from South Africa to England, this was the first time we would be spending any appreciable time apart since our wedding in 1949.

Over the ensuing weeks, months and years, we (and that means the whole family) have been treated with unfailing kindness by staff and volunteers alike. We are never made to feel in the way, no matter what time we visit or phone. And we have gradually come to accept that this is truly B's home now; staff and volunteers – indeed sometimes the relatives of other residents too – have become like a valued extension of our own family. The care and dedication shown has been above and beyond the call of duty. And though I miss him dreadfully, it is very clear to me that we could never have given him the quality of life approaching what the home provides.

As for myself and my new life, there have certainly been difficult adjustments to make. One acquaintance (a man) said to me after we'd met on a number of occasions, 'Now, why did I think you were a widow?' Why indeed? In common with many people in similar situations, one feels 'neither here nor there' in this respect. And it's not a particularly easy or comfortable feeling... But, as I said, one adjusts.

I am still very heavily involved with B's care, with his ever-changing needs, and this brings not only the worry and concern and sadness, but also precious flashes of joy. As a family we have learned to savour these moments of happiness shared with our beloved B. And indeed I feel that we have become even closer as a family as we have gone through the experience together.

I have found my work as a volunteer with the Jewish Care carers' service extremely rewarding, and also find it interesting and worthwhile to involve myself in activities of organisations like Uniting Carers for Dementia.

Spending time with family and friends also goes a long way to 'keeping me sane'.

I must also mention the wonderful contribution made to our wellbeing by the volunteer team who run the regular services at the care home's little synagogue. These occasions afford B obvious satisfaction and pleasure on a deep emotional and spiritual level in these later years of his life, when the pleasure he used to take in good conversation, reading, and so on are beyond his reach. He had had the average 'middle-of-the-road' Jewish boy's upbringing, with a fair amount of religious tradition and exposure to the cultural heritage, and in particular had enjoyed the liturgical musical aspect. But during the years we were married, neither of us had been especially observant of all the religious rules. Our synagogue involvement had been largely centred on the major holy days rather than on weekly Sabbath attendance. Now, however, we were thrilled to become part of this warmly embracing little congregation at its regular weekly service as well as on the holidays. And B revelled in joining in the old remembered blessings and above all the singing that he always loved.

The life of a carer for someone with dementia is many-faceted. It brings stress and great sadness, but it can also include many moments of deep-felt happiness and shared love.[1]

Note

[1]   Since this chapter was written, Debbie's husband has died. Debbie wrote anonymously about her experiences of caring for her husband in the Jewish Care carers' newsletter, *Careline*, issue 53, summer 2007. Names have been changed.

6

$\mathcal{W}$e Learn to Enter her World

U Hla Htay

Origins

My wife Minnie was diagnosed with early onset Alzheimer's dementia in November 1996, at the age of 59. Her behaviour had started to become strange round about 1992, and she had initially been misdiagnosed with depression, and prescribed Prozac. But something was not right, and when our old GP retired, the new GP – whose own mother had dementia – immediately made a referral to the consultant neurologist.

I informed our three sons, then aged 24, 22 and 19, on the same day and told Minnie's brothers, sisters and aunts a week later. Getting our sons involved from the very beginning was my first dilemma: as a father I wanted to protect my sons from feelings which could be distressing, but they did have the right to know their mother's diagnosis. They have been supportive and helpful to Minnie and me ever since. This reduces my burden of caring and stress. The heartwarming feeling of knowing that family support is there whenever needed is always a comfort, and encourages me to give Minnie the best loving care. My sons' partners are also very supportive and give us excellent help.

We started to research what dementia is, thinking about how to prepare and proceed with our individual lives and as a family. We became aware that caring for Minnie would require patience, perseverance and understanding and could be a long-haul process lasting many years.

Minnie is Eurasian, born in Myanmar (Burma) to an Irish father and Shan mother. They were evacuated from Burma during World War II and lived in Bangalore and Kashmir for a few years before moving to Belfast in the late 1950s; they then settled in Northampton. We met in London in 1965, when I was working for the Burmese national shipping line, and got married in

1971. The Burmese ambassador officiated at the wedding and our marriage was blessed by Buddhist monks.

Minnie was a straightforward person, always one to speak her mind, yet polite, warm, charming and fun. She was kind and considerate, loved her three sons equally and would do anything for them. She was firm and fair with her sons and with the children at the local primary school where she worked as a meal supervisor. She cooked, fed us, ironed clothes and cleaned the house, and exercised without fail every night.

Then Minnie's personality changed; she started calling our sons by the wrong names, falling asleep at dinner, getting into disagreements with work colleagues (which she had never done before), and not completing tasks; she lost interest in cooking and domestic tasks; her use of language changed and she stopped exercising. As Minnie was dealing with children, we had to arrange for her to resign from the school.

When her abilities were gradually waning, I felt my heart was being chipped away bit by bit, and I became distraught. This was not good for my health. But now, when I am able to recognise her remaining abilities, however minute, it renews my determination to look after her. My sons constantly check my health and encourage me to look after myself, so that I can really take good care of Minnie.

Trials and tribulations

Our three sons and I agreed after the diagnosis that from now on we must understand that Minnie's actions and behaviour are driven by the disease, not her intention to hurt us in any way, or anyone around us. Thus, although there were initial embarrassments and some difficulties, we accepted her behaviour. We then began to realise that we do not need to excuse her behaviour to the public. At times, members of the public are shocked to witness Minnie's occasional outbursts and assume such behaviour is directed at them personally. They can be unsympathetic, rude and abusive in response. At first I used to try to explain Minnie's condition to those people – some are ready to listen and to understand, others not so. My sons suggested we should leave it to their ignorance.

As we want Minnie to enjoy a normal family life, we go shopping together, walking in public places and in the parks – especially in Regent's Park with its rose garden, to enjoy the swathe of colours and variety of scents with different ground textures. We go to coffee shops and participate in social and cultural events, as long as we are not a nuisance to other people.

Going to the toilet with her was a new challenge for me to face. To avoid the screaming of the ladies, I used to take Minnie to the Gents with me. One could see the suspicious and amused male faces when we came out of the toilet. I then acquired a RADAR key for the use of disabled toilets in public places, but was met by some funny looks from the public. Once when we used a disabled toilet in Regent's Park, the toilet attendant pointed to the wheelchair sign, indicating that it's only for the use of those with a physical disability.

Minnie never used to be disrespectful to anybody, and would never swear or use any foul language. She started referring to me as the 'old man', but this changed to 'you b****rd' and 'you b**ch'. At first I was so annoyed with her and strongly objected, but it would not register with her. When I reacted adversely to her, Minnie's face would fall and she would look at me with the eyes of a doe. Then I reminded myself that she did not mean to hurt or provoke me. I started to ignore it, and just respond with a smile, and this brings peace to us.

One day we were at a cash till, and she started calling me names. In front of me was an Australian gay man, who accused Minnie of being rude to him. On several occasions, old ladies have shied away from us when she displayed such colourful language in public. When shunned for her behaviour, Minnie would say that it was not her but the other woman! (It is true, from her perspective, that it was acted out by the disease not by her *per se*.)

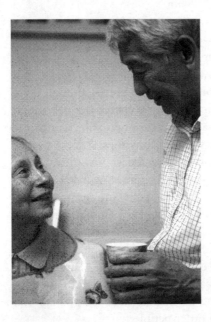

U Hla Htay and his wife Minnie Htay © Alzheimer's Society

In the summer of 2003, we attended a wedding and Minnie was in her element joining in and singing along with the proceedings. I got embarrassed and told her I would never take her to similar occasions. However, I do still take her everywhere when invited, including engagement parties, funerals and embassy receptions. I just need twice the time to get Minnie ready.

Minnie's dementia has affected her speech and choice of words. She says, 'Get away from you!' for 'Keep away from me!' She gets into conversation with the recorded message on the answerphone. She talks to her mother's portrait as if addressing her mother. When advised to do something, Minnie says, 'No, no, no,' when she means, 'Yes, yes, yes,' – like Jim from *The Vicar of Dibley*.

Once we were out together, and Minnie complained to a man on the street that I was following her. The poor man was at a loss whether to help her – he was not at all convinced that I was her husband. We could laugh about it later, but it was trying at the time.

Getting the right treatment and care

Behaviour problems increased in 2001. When a young home respite sitter could not stand any more of Minnie's wanting to listen to Elvis and Dean Martin, a struggle broke out, and Minnie was alleged to have assaulted her. After a thorough investigation by the social services care manager and me, the allegation was dropped.

That summer, because of Minnie's frequent and heightened behaviour problems, a locum consultant psychiatrist prescribed four times above the normal starter dose of the neuroleptic haloperidol. Within twelve hours Minnie was totally slumped in a chair, with no intake of food or drink; after eighteen hours her eyes were glazed and she could not recognise us: she had become like a zombie and the left side of her face had become distorted. We requested the consultant to stop but he insisted he wanted to observe for the next three to five days. We categorically insisted he must stop the medicine. The Admiral nurse gave me information from the British National Formulary (professional guide for prescribing drugs) and an Alzheimer's Society Factsheet[1] which helped us to challenge the consultant. He mentioned that in his country, patients like Minnie would be given electric shock therapy. The mental health nurse accompanying the consultant suggested that to maintain treatment they could section Minnie, which we totally rejected. We said we would make a legal challenge, as Minnie is not a danger to the public or herself. In the end, he agreed to reduce the dosage in steps over three days, supplemented with Aricept. When the permanent consultant psychiatrist was in post, he put Minnie into an assessment unit and dropped the haloperidol.

Later in the year the consultant recommended that Minnie should move into an NHS care home, to which I initially agreed. After discussions with the family, I rescinded my decision and suggested caring for Minnie alternate weeks at home and at the care home, with a review every six months. This arrangement was put in place, but over the years our sons became concerned over my health and wellbeing, and so the respite care has been revised to a one month on/one month off basis. Our quality of life is better when Minnie is at home and it is more convenient for our sons and friends to visit and interact with her. I get more anxious, and my blood pressure is higher, when Minnie is at the respite centre, although at times it is physically and mentally exhausting having her at home. During the month of respite I relax, re-energise and refresh. Sometimes I visit my brother and sister abroad, or do voluntary work.

During her stays at the respite centre, we are always in close communication with the staff to ensure high quality care. We have come across healthcare assistants who have put shoes on the wrong feet; left gloves in her pants; and shaved her eyebrows and pubic hair. Minnie was sexually assaulted by another patient and an overdose of medicine was administered. We had to make an official complaint. We are normally reluctant to make complaints and try to resolve issues at the centre management level, but when they close ranks we are left with no option. At the care homes, there is – to some degree – a culture of acceptance and tolerance by the professionals of sexual transgressions by patients against other patients. With healthcare assistants of various ethnic origins, there are sometimes language and cultural issues. Staff retention is a problem and most of the staff have very little training in dementia care. They sometimes ignore the basic care needs of vulnerable patients with dementia, some of whom do not have active support from their families. We realise that care staff are trying their best in very difficult circumstances, but feel strongly that a radical change of attitude and culture is urgently required.

Accessing support

When Admiral Nurse Services offered monthly support visits in 1997, I thought it was too frequent, and so we had no help initially. Later, I found it really helpful to discuss care strategies, coping mechanisms and how to access healthcare services. Previously I used to arrange with our three sons to sit with Minnie when I had to go out, and encourage them to attend to her personal care. Later, as they became busier and less available, I realised (with their gentle prompting) that I could access social services and voluntary respite care sitting services, and this began in 2000.

I joined the Alzheimer's Society straight away. The tips and hints and articles by carers about their experiences in the monthly magazine have helped me in caring for Minnie at home, supported by the Society's Factsheets. I pass these on to my sons.

I also give talks on my experience as a carer at *for dementia* and on a mental health nurses course at King's College. Admiral nurses also run a carers' support group where we share our experience of caring for loved ones at home, care strategies, accessing other services, good and bad effects of dementia medicines, accessibility of dementia drugs and so on. This led me to found a Westminster Alzheimer's Café group in 2000, meeting once a month for people with dementia and their carers with the help of an Admiral nurse. As music is an excellent stimulation for people with dementia, live musicians are invited on alternate months. Learning from other family carers is inspirational and helps my day-to-day caring strategy.

The right way to eat Peking duck

Dementia carers have to face ethical issues all the time. We can only act in all good faith and love, but we can never know whether what we did was the right thing to do. We have to take comfort in the fact that we have tried to act in the best interests of the person with dementia (at the same time, recognising that there may have been some element of our own personal choice as well).

When Minnie says she wants to go to her mum's place, she will not accept the explanation that her mother died some 40 years ago. Then we put the photo of her mother in the room and whenever Minnie asks for her, we point to the photo, and that settles her. At times, Minnie calls me by the name of her elder brother and gets upset when I correct her.

In the summer of 2001, the wake of a friend was celebrated at a Chinese restaurant and Peking duck was served. People at the table proceeded to serve the meal in the traditional way, but Minnie would not accept it. We had to mix all the ingredients of the dish together – only then would Minnie eat it.

Through these caring experiences we learn to enter her world, rather than insist on her joining ours. Going with the flow with Minnie is less stressful for both of us, and no harm is done. Sometimes, with a person with dementia, reality checks can bring adverse effects to the carer and the cared-for.

Spirituality

I am a Buddhist, and meditate regularly. In the earlier days, Minnie would keep herself busy washing the dishes, or polishing. Then her shouting started. When asked to keep the noise down, she stayed quiet for a few minutes but then it would start all over again. Then Minnie began to sit by me, either talking or falling asleep. At one time, Minnie was so fascinated by hats that she would put one on me and, tapping my shoulder, she would say, 'You look so nice, I like you.' Or she would tap my shoulder and ask whether I love her, and if so to nod. This annoyed me enormously at first, because it distracted me from my meditation. Later it cracked me up with laughter and I would end up hugging her.

I look on the ups and downs of daily care as challenges, and when I reflect upon them, they become less of a burden. It becomes a joy to carry on caring for Minnie and learn new coping strategies. When a caring intervention is just

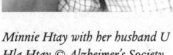

Minnie Htay with her husband U Hla Htay © Alzheimer's Society

right, and Minnie gives me a smile or a word of appreciation, all the frustrations and bad feelings disappear and it makes my day.

Hopes and wishes

As Minnie now has very little verbal communication, we have to be more vigilant, and observe her behaviour minutely so as to interpret her needs and to find ways of stimulating her senses. When Minnie sees us, her eyes light up with a faint smile and at times with a few words of greeting. She has become more tactile, and always appreciates a hug and a kiss on the cheek. Our sons used to address her as 'Mum' but now she only responds to her name, so they now address her by her name, as I do.

In the last couple of years, two of my sons have got married and we have now become grandparents. Minnie has attended the weddings with us, as we would not let her miss such joyous family celebrations. We very much appreciate the understanding and generous support afforded to us by our in-laws and friends. These occasions were really enjoyable and it was heartwarming to see Minnie dancing away the night.

When I see elderly couples I wish I could be like them with Minnie – sharing jokes, family affairs, enjoying things we used to enjoy. My comforting thought is that we are giving her all our love and care, and that Minnie knows and appreciates this. We are determined to look after Minnie as long as we can, to give her happiness and comfort in the years to come.

Note

1   See Alzheimer's Society (2008) *Factsheet 408: Dementia: Drugs used to Relieve Depression and Behavioural Symptoms.* (Available at www.alzheimers.org.uk/factsheet/408, accessed 20 March 2009.)

7

Half a World Away

Anna Young

October 2007: Aqua Calientes, Peru

I can't believe all I've done in the last few days. I've climbed, scrambled, been hauled up and down to see some of the most sacred sites in Peru, a country I've always wanted to visit since a friend sent me a blurry black and white postcard from there nearly twenty years ago. Three years ago, when I planned this trip, I broke my leg. Then two years ago another trip was cancelled. Now I'm here. We've been very active, but amazingly I don't hurt anywhere. I've ached more after a day in the garden! It makes me realise how much of me I have put into caring for and about Crispian. I have willed him to get better. I have hoped that by caring for him in the best way possible he might stabilise. I have wept many tears, shouted to the listening air, frightened him with my oaths at three in the morning, when I'm changing sheets for the second time that night.

To no avail. Every day, no matter how I care, or what I do, he has slipped, even tumbled. (Literally sometimes, as when he fell on to a large plant pot full of geraniums, and gashed his hand.) He is leaving me behind. I don't know where he is going, and I don't understand the language, or the country wherein he dwells. Try as hard as I may to pull him back from the edge of the abyss called dementia, he is leaving me anyway.

I hold him for a moment, sometimes for up to an hour, with quizzes, crosswords, memory games. He says in moments of crystal lucidity, 'Why is this happening? What's wrong, why can't I think properly, why do I lose my way?'

I tell him it's the illness. This always seems to soothe him. It's not him, I tell him, it's his brain. Spectacularly, once, after I'd screamed at him for some perceived misdemeanour, I told him that it wasn't him I was mad at, but the illness. Twenty-four hours later, he said, 'You know when you said it wasn't me you were mad with, but the illness?'

'Yes,' I replied, waiting expectantly for a criticism.

'Well,' he continued, 'I found that really helpful.'

January 2008

This morning the home rang me. He had had a nose bleed (the fourth this week) and a fall at 3 a.m. Thank God they didn't ring me. He had been unconscious for some minutes. They called the paramedics and today he has sore ribs. The manager said that he didn't think that Crispian's ribs were broken but bruised and that he would keep his eye on him. Why did he fall at 3 a.m.? Why wasn't he fast asleep? The staff at the home have told me that he wanders about in the night, and since he retires at about 7.15 p.m. (because he is exhausted by then, and falls asleep in his chair, so they get him to bed), he probably wakes at 2 or 3 a.m. having slept his requirements.

What will happen? How will this end – because end it will: how far away is the day when someone will ring me and tell me that he has had a heart attack, or a bad fall, or has pneumonia? Would it help if I knew? We all

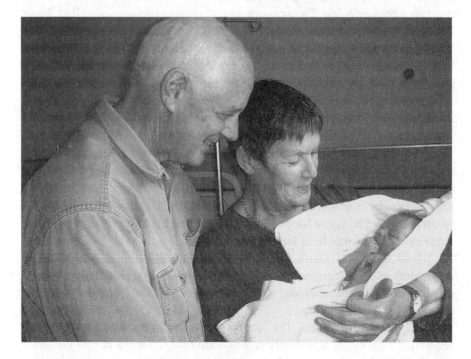

Crispian and Anna in 2003 with grandson Lev

agree in the family that he has some quality of life; he loves us and his family, especially the grandchildren, and is delighted and proud when we visit him. He loves all visitors, and is visibly pleased to see them. He loves going out for a stroll, when he will sometimes walk unaided, then begin to bend over, and stagger, and needs to go in his wheelchair. Sometimes, when he is wobbly on his feet, and unable to walk at all, we just visit him at the home in one of the lounges, where we are brought tea and biscuits by the staff.

We talk, or rather he talks, and we try and guess the context of his conversation. Only people close to him, who know his life history, can begin to hazard a guess at what he might be talking about. For example, one day the staff witnessed him getting his suitcase from his room, lug it to the lounge, and sit on a chair. When asked what he was doing, he replied, 'I'm waiting for the train, and I can't leave the platform in case the train comes.' He became anxious when they tried to change the situation. He sat there for hours evidently.

When I visited him later in the day, I gently told him of the staff's concerns, and reminded him of his actions. He replied, 'I was waiting for the train.' I asked him where he was going on the train, and he replied, 'To school.' It all made sense. From the age of nine years he boarded at a minor public school. He would sometimes have to take himself back to school after the holidays. His mother would drive him to the local station, and put him on the platform with instructions not to move, and the guard would have to make sure he got on to the right train, and a member of the school's staff would meet him off the train. It all made sense (if you knew the context). It is sad that the home does not have enough staff, so there was not time for one of them to sit and talk with him. They could have had an interesting conversation and the member of staff could have heard how children of nine or ten were entrusted to the railways in the late 1940s!

January 2008

I spend half my time feeling fiercely protective of him, wanting to be with him all the time, like a guardian angel, watching him, making sure those that care for him do it compassionately and intelligently; the other half of me wants him dead. Isn't that a dreadful thing to say, to write, to see in print?

I spoke to a friend the other day. Her husband had died suddenly; he was ill for a week and she and the family knew, for a week, that he was going to die. She told me that she and her children were able to hold him and say goodbye to him. She remarked that with Crispian's illness, he is dying slowly, and I say goodbye to him emotionally every day. At the group I attend, one of the women refers to dementia as 'a journey'. I call it a death sentence. You don't recover, you die from it. It's hardly a journey one undertakes – and if it is a journey, then it is one he has been hijacked on to, as though a black coach has come steaming out of the night and a highwayman has scooped him up and tied him to the top of the coach and the horses have galloped off with him into the darkness.

If he were dead, we could close the book and move on, move away. I would buy a studio flat in Marrakech. We would remember him with love and laughter. This way, we remember him with resentment, anger, anguish, sadness – and frustration with the system that does not, cannot help us. He was always a prudent, caring man, saved, put money away for the future and the children. We did not have expensive holidays; we took a caravan to France or, amazingly one year, to Spain. Now we have to spend the money on his care, and even pay tax for the privilege. It is not his fault. It happened. Dementia happened.

Even when we talk, there is an increasing distance between us, as though he is drifting further and further away from me and our relationship – which of course he is. I no longer recognise the man in front of me. Is this the man I have shared my life with for the last 40 years? Seeing the film *Malcolm and Barbara*[1] enabled me to make the decision that I could not do what Barbara did and care for my husband unto the end. There is not enough of me. We need six of me to do this job.

Last year I lost five stone in weight. The timing is propitious although I have not been able to work out why it is so. At a time when I need to be more of me, certainly in spirit, I became smaller in body, deliberately. I found a diet that worked for me, for the first time in my life. When I weighed 16 stone, and he fell over, I could at least turn him with my foot. Now 11 stone, I could barely move him at all, and had to leave him there, which necessitated me getting help to move him. Perhaps it was this act that made me realise that I needed help. Couldn't do the job on my own. Capable all my life, strong, resilient, an organiser, suddenly admitting defeat. The person I loved most defeated me.

February 2008

Today I went to view an apartment. The thought of moving both scares and excites me. We have been here 25 years, but the maintenance of this house is getting hard for me. There is always something to do, the trees, the garden, the drains. It seems that every time I step outside I notice something else that needs doing. Although I have family nearby, I also know that they are very busy with their own young families.

I think Crispian enjoyed his time out, being wheeled along the seafront. It's hard to tell. I needed to get something from the boot and left him in the passenger seat, and suddenly the car was moving forward. I leaped towards the driver's seat, and by that time he had put the handbrake back on again! I put my head down on the steering wheel and wept. I said to him through clenched teeth, 'You put the handbrake off!'

He said, 'Yes, but I put it back on again!'

When we got upstairs, we had the usual wrestle while I tried to take his jacket off, his arms stiffening as I slid the arms of the garment from his arms. I know what I ought to do. I ought to explain slowly and carefully what my actions are to be, then assist him gently with the action. Given what had just happened and the thought that we could have slid gently into the main road, or the wall, what's best to do deserts me at times like these.

Caring for Crispian breaks my heart and at the same time, hardens it. I have so much compassion for him and his condition. A part of him is aware of what is happening to him. After the handbrake incident, and when I was leaving, he said, 'It's not working out, is it?' I repeated his words to him, and asked what's not working out. He replied 'You, me, the children, their children...' His voice trailed off. I think that he was aware that I had been cross with him and that he had upset me, and I think this tied in with his previous marriage that ended in divorce (40 years ago). In his head, time and space are fused, thoughts and ideas don't follow a logical pathway. The neurologist explained that clumps of brain cells are dying in his brain, so that when he has an idea or thought, the thought has to jump over the clump and, of course, who knows where it will land. Sometimes, he can hear himself make the illogical jump, and will laugh, and say, 'I don't know where I'm going with this!' When he says something like this I find it so poignant. This oh-so-intelligent man knows that his intellect is crumbling away.

February 2008

Today when I woke up I wanted to be somewhere else. But as usual, I will struggle with the wheelchair again, pushing and shoving it into the boot of the car, along with the seat, the bag, the hat and gloves, the nappy bag with spare pads and wipes, and go and collect him from the home. We will go down to the seaside, and he will stumble and fall or walk off in the opposite direction, and not be able to see the wheelchair, and when he sees the wheelchair he will be unable to sit down on the seat. My daughter and I encourage him to bend his knees to enable him to sit, but he resolutely refuses, and we repeat, 'Bend your knees, bend your knees,' until he understands. We eat out in a very tolerant-staffed restaurant; we blunder in off the seafront, buggies, toddlers, four-year-olds, the wheelchair, all the anoraks, blankets, and so on that we need for a blustery cold day in February. It takes ages to get him up out of the wheelchair and into a chair at a table. I pray that he went to the loo before he left the home, because I can't bear the thought of taking him there when it isn't a disabled loo, as there won't be enough room for me to help him relieve himself. If all this sounds heartless and resentful, it's because I don't know where my heart in relation to him has gone. This man I loved so deeply and for so long, with whom I brought up five children, is transformed into some person I no longer recognise.

This is not a job I would voluntarily do. I am resentful – resentful that this is our retirement, that I am awaiting a major operation, and that it's all turned out so differently.

October 2007: Machu Picchu

It's the end of October and I'm hotter here in the sun than I have been all summer in UK. Crispian is in a care home. I'm here in Peru. It's bizarre. Last week he was convinced that I was going to divorce him and he told the care staff, so they told me when I arrived to take him home for the day. No matter how I assured him that after 38 years of marriage I had no intention of divorcing him, he remained convinced and fretted about 'what to tell the children'. When I asked him about his thinking, he said, 'Well, it's the logical conclusion, isn't it? I'm here in this hotel, you're there. We're separated. It's the next step.' The care staff had listened to his complaints that there were no double rooms, so it wasn't possible for me to go and live there, too. He worries that we may have to sell the house so that we may continue to pay for the 'hotel'. When he talks, I have to unscramble the meaning. It's as though the words and meaning are all there but all jumbled up. If I remain calm, I try to get the possible context; it's all guesswork, like a cryptic crossword. You go along with a supposed context, and also his accompanying mood – anxious, jolly, serene, playful, and so on. Then halfway through the process, giving him feedback on which to test my hypothesis, he suddenly looks tired and frustrated and says, 'No, it's not that.' So on I go (patience is a necessary part of this decoding process), testing another possible context. This can take up to three times longer than it took for him to make his initial utterance. But if he smiles, and says, 'Yes, yes, that's it,' I am encouraged, and can proceed to decipher. If I 'get it right', he is so pleased, and for a treasured moment, we are on the same wavelength. I don't think too hard about this, because the implications of being on the same wavelength, and the amount of persistence, energy and patience this takes, is in contrast to the relationship we had for most of 38 years. We focused on rearing five children; we would finish each other's sentences, and just a look or a sigh would convey to the other a whole panoply of meanings and emotions. I am, as I write this, by the Amazon river; buses going up to Machu Picchu, hens clucking around my feet, in contrast to the smart hotels over the road, half a world away.

That strikes me as being a good title for this piece, because we are half a world away in relationship, whilst we both struggle with this illness that deprives us of so much. Maybe I have to be half a world away physically to reach an emotional independence. As I am travelling alone, I can write detachedly and connectedly about the process of dementia in relationship.

The carer has a resurgence of brain activity, as new thinking is required to cope with the burden of dementia in a relationship. There is a coming together, if one enters into a symbiosis with the sufferer. If the carer supplies every need of the demented person, she then has to diminish her own needs. It is not possible for two to survive in this relationship without some massive realignment of the boundaries. The re-thinking or re-definition that is required takes enormous energy, as the carer's needs are superseded by the needs of the sufferer. Even if it has been an equal relationship, the carer becomes the controller of the other: necessary, because otherwise *the dementia controls*. The dementia is not the person.

So there is by definition a separation, and a struggle by the non-afflicted to see the person, the essence, and not his controller: his atrophying brain. We need to remember we are of the same world, we occupy the same space. And there is the struggle, daily, to remember who he is, and who I am, and who we were, and who we are.[2]

Notes

1   Paul Watson's film *Malcolm and Barbara: Love's Farewell* shown on ITV in 2007. See also Chapter 28 of this book, 'When Words Fail'.

2   Crispian died peacefully on 22 April 2009.

Have You Seen my Pat?

Pat Hill

My husband has an unusual dementia, which the doctors at the National Hospital for Neurology and Neurosurgery at Queen Square, London have been unable to fully diagnose. It may be related to Alzheimer's, but it doesn't fit a normal pattern. Something called prosopagnosia was mentioned by the consultant psychiatrist: an inability to recognise faces and places. They would like Derrick's brain to be donated to the Queen Square brain bank after his death.

Derrick and I were married in 1957 and have now celebrated our golden wedding. He was born in Bootle in 1930, but his family moved to Southport after all the windows and the door of their house were blown out in the bombing. He did his national service in the navy, and afterwards trained as a navigator in the RAF, and served in coastal command. After leaving the RAF, he worked for 34 years as a sales rep for Rowntree Mackintosh. Whilst at work, he studied with the Open University, and gained an upper second Honours degree. He loved reading, and our bedrooms were lined with books.

Derrick first had periods of feeling nauseous and giddy in 1996, aged 66. It would occur about every eight weeks. He would feel sick several times during a 24-hour period, with a strange feeling in his nose and mouth, and a strange taste. Tests showed he was likely to have a form of epilepsy. However, I have never seen Derrick have a fit. He did run into the back of someone's car for no apparent reason about this time, so he was told to surrender his driving licence. Over the next few years, Derrick was given many drugs for epilepsy: he became a shaking, dribbling, gaunt wreck as they tried every drug they could think of – some for weeks and others only for days. Nothing seemed to help.

Derrick was referred to our local community mental health team for older people. The consultant psychiatrist and the nurses in the unit saw Derrick and me constantly, but Derrick refused to go to any day care centres. He would just walk out. I was able to take Derrick to the monthly Maidstone Alzheimer's tea party and outings for a while, and they have continued to be there for me over the years.

When Derrick became very difficult, I also had a monthly visit from an Admiral nurse who has always given me lots of support and advice. She helped me fill in forms and came round looking at nursing homes with me. She suggested I took Derrick into a family changing room when we went swimming, so I wouldn't keep losing him. She also encouraged me to buy a key for disabled toilets, so that I could go in with Derrick and change him if necessary. They are always there to listen to my troubles. I've been very lucky.

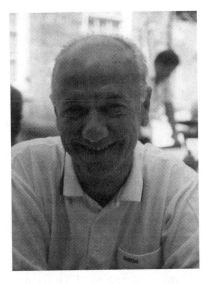

Derrick, c.1989

Over the years, Derrick became more confused, and began to think I was about sixteen different people. In his eyes, I would change several times a day into different people: I've been French, Japanese, Chinese, men, women, assorted female relations and nurses – but then, desperate to find the real me, he'd be knocking up the neighbours at night, saying, 'Have you seen my Pat?' He'd be ringing the police at all hours, saying I'd been abducted. He did this five times. He was really upset, because I had supposedly gone off with my brother-in-law. He was screaming down the phone to send me back. He couldn't accept the fact that I was right there beside him – he just thought I was his sister, Dorothy. He became fed up with all the 'strangers' in the house.

One day I found a hammer by the bed which Derrick had put there to protect himself. I had to hide it, and from then on the psychiatrist made me promise to leave the house if Derrick thought I was a stranger and ordered me out. One night I refused to leave, and he got his arm round my neck and dragged me up the road in the pouring rain, in my slippers. He said, 'A very nice lady will take you in. You're not staying with me!' He knocked on my friend's door, and after a cup of tea, she was able to convince him that I was Pat.

Another night, at 2.30 a.m., after he had spent hours ringing round trying to find me, he noticed the emerald ring on my finger (a twentieth anniversary gift), and, not recognising me, he said I'd stolen it from Pat. He fetched a pair of scissors, a cheese knife and a skewer from the kitchen drawer, and told me he wanted Pat's ring back. I thought I might lose my finger! It was very tight, but fortunately I managed to get it off with washing up liquid. He said I had to leave, but then he noticed my handbag, and said, 'You've stolen her handbag, too!' and took it from me. This meant I had no keys, or money, or mobile – they were all in the bag. Out into the night I went, wondering what to do. Suddenly I saw my neighbour's lights were on. She'd come down for a coffee and a doughnut at 2.45, and she cheerfully invited me in. I am so thankful for my friends. It seemed like a miracle, finding someone up in my hour of need.

Derrick used to ask me to leave almost daily. I used to keep blouses and pretty scarves in neighbours' houses so as to change my appearance. I would leave by the back door, and then phone on the mobile and say I was his wife Pat, and would he like me to come home. He'd say, 'Oh, yes, please, I've had an awful woman here!' I'd change clothes, put some lipstick on and appear at the front door. I soon realised that if I left by the back door without saying goodbye, and appeared at the front door later, he would sometimes start looking for the 'other' me, supposedly still in the house, to introduce me! He also commented that people were very rude, and that they would come and visit and not have the courtesy to say goodbye and thank you. After that I always said goodbye, and assured him that he'd soon be seeing Pat. This worked better.

One awful Christmas, he ordered our son Jon, his wife and their toddler, Jessica, out of the house. He didn't know them. I had to phone a hotel, which fortunately had a room. It was pouring and dark, and little Jessica was crying. So was I, as I stood in the rain and saw them off. The next morning they phoned and said could they come back for a few hours. I told Derrick they were coming to visit and he greeted them with open arms! He had no knowledge of the night before.

Derrick refused to stay at the various groups that had been organised, which would have given me a break. I was eventually allowed a couple of two-hour sessions with someone from Crossroads sitting with Derrick so I could shop and go swimming. Sometimes he wouldn't let me drive the car when he didn't recognise me. He said I wasn't insured. It made it very difficult if I had an appointment. He is very strong, so I didn't want a wrestling match. Derrick had never been violent, and we had a very happy marriage, so I felt tearful if he tried to punch me.

Derrick once told the nurse who visited us that he kept finding strange women in his bed, and a couple of times he did say perhaps I should sleep somewhere else, as he really wanted his Pat, and not someone he didn't know.

Eventually, Derrick didn't recognise our house. He would crouch by the front door, begging to be taken home. I would drive him right round Maidstone, and then hope he would recognise our home when we returned. Sometimes, Derrick couldn't find our bedroom. He'd be curled up on the floor, or downstairs, lost. I labelled the doors. It didn't help. I deadlocked the outer doors: he climbed out of the window, over the sink unit, ripping the nets and bringing down the window box and its metal supports. During the last few weeks before he went away, he washed his face down the toilet and messed on the carpet and trod it all over the house.

The drugs were making Derrick very woozy at night and if he went down on the floor, I couldn't lift him. I had to call the ambulance two nights running. So he went in for respite care, but while he was there, he had a fall, which crushed one of his vertebrae. He spent ten weeks in hospital, and I was told he would never walk again. At that point, in June 2004, he was admitted to a very good nursing home for the elderly mentally infirm.

He used to bite and punch the staff, sometimes, when they were changing him. But he was usually okay with me, if he knew I was Pat. Most of his speech is now unintelligible. Sometimes a sentence does come out the right way up – almost as if loose wires have reconnected briefly.

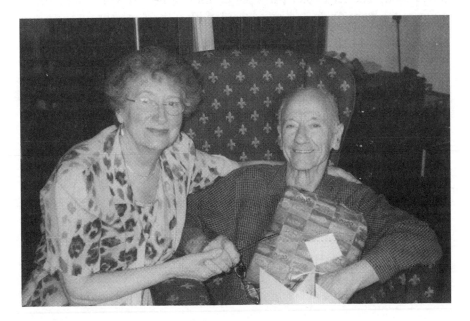

Pat with Derrick on his birthday, 2004

He is largely incontinent. He used to feel he shouldn't wet himself, but he could no longer tell anyone the problem. If he wasn't watched every minute, on different occasions, he pulled down his pad and peed in plant pots, on the table, in someone's basket of soft toys, over chairs, up the wall, and, most dangerously, on the TV screen. He was hastily turned to one side in case he electrocuted himself! He has now passed this stage and is changed regularly.

He is always fiddling with things. He ripped a door off his new wardrobe. Fortunately the home has a very good handyman, who is constantly being called upon to repair various items. The next time Derrick tried to rip the door off, the whole wardrobe tipped forward. The contents of the top shelf and the items stored on top all hit a nurse on the head, and the poor girl was under the wardrobe. Derrick burst out laughing. Fortunately they had managed to push him to one side as it tipped. It's now bolted to the wall.

Derrick had a hip replacement in 2006. I constantly had to remind staff in the orthopaedic ward about his dementia. Soluble paracetamol, still in foil, would be put in front of him, and would still be there hours later. A liquid laxative, left for him in a small container, he rubbed on his head. He got very sticky, and it didn't help his constipation. He couldn't take foil lids off orange juice, or deal with butter wrapped in foil. On being given a three-course meal all on one tray, Derrick happily tipped the soup on the main course and added cherry cheesecake on top. He seemed to enjoy it. I did ask if he could have a little dignity, and have some pants put on him, as he was lying with nothing on from the waist down in a mixed ward, with visitors present.

Derrick surprised everyone, because he did eventually learn to walk again after returning to the home, though he is bent right over, and hanging on to the furniture, and has to have morphine up to four times a day to help with the pain in his back and hip. All drugs for epilepsy have been stopped, and he seems better off without them as he no longer dribbles.

I take old catalogues to the home, so that Derrick can turn the pages and happily rip a few out. It keeps him occupied for a while. I noticed Derrick was looking at a book recently, and it was upside down. Then he chewed the corner. To think that Derrick used to get cross, all those years ago, if he saw someone turn down the corners of a book.

The Open University still send correspondence addressed to Derrick. The latest asked if he'd be interested in taking a postgraduate course which might further his career.

Derrick eats well. He does not seem unhappy. I have no idea how many years we still have. I am thankful that I have a good family and friends. I still love Derrick, and for a minute or two each day, he knows that I'm his Pat.

9

Feisty Love

Maria Smith

We've suffered a robbery:
the most vile, cowardly steal.
Silently, invisibly, impalpably,
the thief fled our lives,
leaving behind
a trail of destruction,
deprivation,
desperation and dislocations,
indifferent to all sufferings,
unmoved by our sorrow.

He was identified as Alzheimer's,
but the stolen property
was not returned,
the damage never repaired.

This thief lifted
Lonnie's memory and cognition
out of his life.
An insidious dismantling of his skills
followed.
Out went most of his meaningful speech.
His coordination faltered,
balance wavered.
Strange paranoias surfaced.
The ability to make choices
a thing of the past.
Cause and effect
became unhinged.

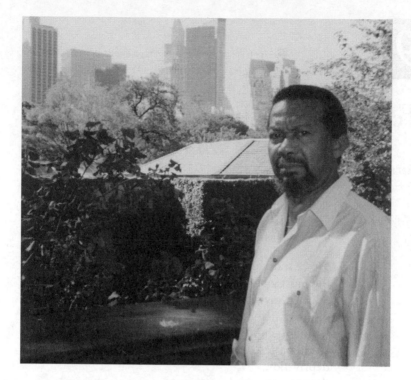

Lonnie in New York, 2000

And so it was
that
all of our lives suffered
a 9/11 type of event.

For him,
a life's worth of memories
crumbled and pulverised
on impact with Alzheimer's.
For us, the family,
the reality of our daily lives
became one of
fragmented relationships,
rare and hurried get-togethers.
Pleasures were lost
through missed pivotal events
in the lives of the children
and the grandchildren.

Friendships ceased to grow,
starved as they were
of shared experiences.

Ten years on,
Lonnie sits in his chair
each and every day,
telling me nothing of the world he inhabits.

I, myself, feel bereft
of affection,
attention and companionship.
I look back and see
years of toiling
without feedback;
the here and now
full of soliloquies,
not of the Shakespearean kind:
there are no audiences, no applause.
The soul feels fractured;
tiredness and anxiety are constant companions.

Only my spirit bounces against the hard rock of despair
and rises
each morning
to face the new day,
determined to make a difference.
I'd like to grow a memorial garden
where our lives together once stood:
I'd celebrate our good times
with a vibrant bed of red tulips;
lay down all unresolved conflicts
and unanswered questions
on a thick patch
of calming lavender.

All grief
dies here.
Feisty love
the only brave survivor.

10

Glimpses of Glory on a Long, Grey Road

Helen Robinson

When I realised that my husband, Chris, had Alzheimer's disease it was as if a great burden had been laid upon my heart and I felt alone and helpless. I was a nurse and for some years I had been involved with Alzheimer's disease, so I knew something of what lay ahead.

We had been married for over 40 years and we loved each other very much. We had supported each other through all the ups and downs of life, but now he seemed to be slipping into a strange world of his own, far from me. He was a preacher, and his robust style of preaching and clarity of thought meant that people from all walks of life had come to hear him preach and to learn about the Bible from him. I found it hard to think that this ability would leave him. As the days passed, a veil of sadness came over everything in my life as I watched the man I loved slowly change.

Through all the six years of his illness there were many who helped us, professional people as well as family and friends. These were some of the glimpses of glory along the grey road, which I remember with gratitude.

I first noticed something strange in Chris's behaviour when he was 65. One day when we were in our usual shopping centre he became completely disorientated. He did not know where he was or which way to go and he did not recover his mental balance till we were driving home. For some time before this he had been forgetful, and his habit of losing things bothered us both, but as he was taking medication for mild epilepsy I thought this could be the cause. He had worked as a chaplain in several prisons and he would often repeat the same prison story to anyone who would care to listen. I found this repetitiveness difficult and boring, not realising that it could be one of the first symptoms of dementia. Perhaps I was in denial.

But that day in the shopping centre was different, and I knew that the alarm bells ringing in my head had to be taken seriously.

Chris and I were both born in Northern Ireland; he came from Belfast and I was a country girl from County Down. We moved to the south of Ireland when we married, as Chris felt God had called him to preach there. We had four children, two boys and two girls, and I was glad that they were around and were adults when Chris was ill.

Chris's faith in God was firm, and when mine was shaky he would say, 'God doesn't make mistakes.' All through his illness he never questioned God or complained against him, though at times he would become frustrated at his inability to remember parts of the Bible, once so familiar to him. The help that I offered only made him more frustrated. I think he was confused about exactly what he was trying to remember.

After that occasion in the shopping centre we went to visit our GP. He talked with us honestly and it was arranged for Chris to visit a specialist in geriatric dementia. Things moved speedily and I felt great relief when Chris was referred to the 'hospital for the elderly'. Here he was assessed and checked in every area. His brain scan confirmed my fears, and the consultant told me that it was Alzheimer's disease. He also told me that one of the significant symptoms of Alzheimer's disease is the patient's ability to 'bluff', and to put on a show of normality.

This was Chris all right! He would pretend that he knew who people were when he hadn't a clue. When someone rang the doorbell he would insist on going to the door. No matter who was there he always called out to me, 'Your friend is at the door for you,' but then it seemed he didn't know what to do next. It seemed as if his train of thought was interrupted and then lost, and I could sense the little tangles in his brain doing their ugly work.

Those visits to the hospital for the elderly helped to take some of the fear and uncertainty from my mind. Every four months we both spent the morning there and received the best of care from a team of different professionals. Best of all, there was a lovely lunch served to the patients. I went to a nearby pub and had lunch and a welcome break. It felt good to be part of a team.

When we married, Chris and I agreed that we would always be honest with each other, and so I believed that it was right to be honest about his illness. When he asked why he couldn't do simple things, and why his memory was 'going to pot', I told him the truth as gently as I could, that he had Alzheimer's disease but that there was help available and he would be given it. He accepted this and I didn't repeat it often.

I think the early days of Chris's illness were more difficult than when the Alzheimer's was more advanced. My diary reminds me of the sadness. I wrote, 'Chris announced today, "My life is very hard."' I had never heard

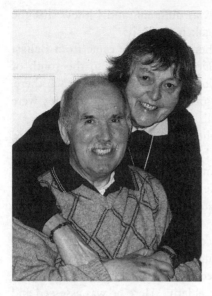

Helen and Chris, when Helen was caring for Chris at home

him say that before and when I asked him to tell me why, he could say nothing more. He suddenly seemed very vulnerable, like a child needing protection, and I felt so helpless to make it better for him. There was anger too in those early days when in the middle of the night he would insist that we should go to our local shop. I would try to reason with him and both of us would end up shouting so loudly I feared we would waken the neighbours.

I became very tired as I lifted him in and out of bed single-handed and I seemed to be constantly helping him to the toilet. My journal records, 'I am so tired, ragged and guilty.'

Having him ready in time and bringing him to church on Sunday morning was difficult. This had been the pattern of his life and it was important to him. It hurt me to see this man who had once been a robust preacher now sitting in the back row picking the threads off his hat. I felt angry that so few people talked to him or even acknowledged his presence. I was comforted by the few who did talk to him with dignity and sincerity. The leader of the choir in our church arranged for members of the choir to come to sing for Chris both at home and later when he was in care. He enjoyed this so much and even though he could not follow all the words he joined in heartily here and there.

Early one Sunday morning Chris woke me with urgent instructions: 'Come on, we had better hurry up or we will be late.'

Thinking that it was a passing notion, I answered him, 'Yes, I will be ready soon. Where are we going?'

He was most insistent. 'To preach to the farmers. Now don't keep us late.'

I asked him to tell me which farmers, but he could not tell me and he was getting cross and frustrated because I was not going fast enough. I got up and dressed us both. We ate some sort of breakfast and then I waited to see what would happen. This man was going somewhere and he was in a hurry! He seemed to have known it was Sunday as soon as he awoke, but as a rule he never knew the days of the week. He fussed us out to the car and I settled him into his seat.

'Where will I go?' I asked, to which he replied insistently, 'To preach to the farmers, go south.'

I began to drive towards the sea and he seemed happy as long as I did not ask him too many questions. When I asked him what he was going to preach about or if he would like me to sing a solo he became angry, so we drove on in silence. When I suggested we choose a hymn for the service he agreed and seemed pleased. One of his favourite hymns was chosen and I began to sing:

My chains fell off, my heart was free,
I rose, went forth, and followed Thee.

Sadness and joy were there in my heart that morning. In all the frustration of his poor confused mind, was his heart free in God's love? I like to think it was.

We never arrived with those farmers, though we drove for many miles. Somehow I managed to turn around towards Dublin and home, and he calmly announced, 'I see we are going back to Dublin.'

When I thought about this episode, I remembered that the first church where he used to preach after we were married was in the country, and most of the congregation were farmers. He was visiting his past memories in the only way he could.

Travelling far was difficult and I found it caused a lot of stress. Often in airports or stations he would wander off if I did not hold on to him continually. We had five grandchildren and he loved them, but as they all lived in England we didn't see them as often as we would have liked. Children seemed able to accept his unpredictable behaviour and being around them made him happy and more relaxed. I had made him a little beanbag for throwing and he was still a fair shot and could cheat well too. He thought that was fun!

I developed a frozen shoulder and lifting Chris was causing me a lot of pain. I visited our GP and straight away he rescued me! He arranged for the public health nurse to call and assess our situation. I found her a great support and for several years she stood by us. She arranged for us to receive all the equipment so necessary for the care of a person with dementia, and also helped with application forms for home care assistance. Being Chris's sole carer was becoming very difficult for me, even though I had help from family and friends.

Chris attended several day care centres each week. He loved being with people but he could be very stubborn and at first he refused to get out of the car and go in.

'You can go in if you want to,' he shouted at me. 'I am not going in.'

After three visits he finally gave in and he ended up loving day care and all the attention and expert care that he received. I appreciated those days of freedom and respite, later to be extended to overnight stays.

Our house became like a nursing home, full of activity. At the centre were two people trying to maintain some semblance of normality. There was a candle on the dinner table and pretty napkins also. Soft music played in the background but there was little conversation. Our worlds were different. Was he lonely? I wondered. There were times when I felt overwhelmed by a sense of loneliness.

There were home carers too. I shall always remember the first one who came.

Eric was a vet from Zimbabwe who was studying here. He worked as a carer to pay his fees and he was all that a carer should be. Chris loved him and they got on well together. In my diary I record, 'Red letter day. Chris allowed Eric to shower him.' Eric finally had to move on and we felt the loss greatly.

Carers came and went, and the road seemed to be unending and very grey. Funds would not cover night care and the nights were becoming a nightmare! I found it hard to sleep and though we had been provided with an electric bed with side guards, Chris could manage to wriggle down to the end and get out. He was incontinent and his general condition was deteriorating. He had developed a habit of spitting out, and meals were becoming a trial of patience for us both.

Sometimes I walked our dog in the grounds of a nearby hospital which was well known for its excellent care of elderly and disabled patients, including those with Alzheimer's. I put Chris's name on the long waiting list, thinking that perhaps one day he would get to the top of the list. I knew that he would receive the best of care there, and as he was very friendly I felt he would be happy to be with other people.

I prayed as I walked with the dog, 'Lord, maybe you would have a place for Chris here some day.' I wasn't pushing it, and I dared not hope, when I thought of that long list. Six months later the phone rang. The doctor in charge was going to come and assess Chris for possible admission.

When she discovered that by now he could barely walk, she announced that they would give him a bed in the long-stay ward as soon as possible. My heart stopped for a moment! Two weeks later, he was offered a place. I find it hard here to describe my feelings. I only know that as I write this, tears are streaming down my face.

What had I done? Was I sending my beloved husband away from me in his time of need? But I knew that he needed more care than I was able to give

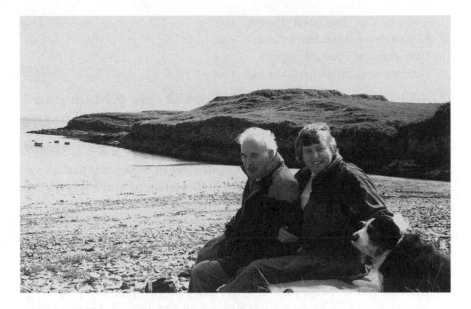

Chris and Helen with their dog Sally in Donegal

him, and now I must accept the sad fact that he had left us some time ago. He was in the strange world of the Alzheimer's patient.

On 15 May 2004 Chris was admitted to the long-stay ward. That day will be imprinted on my mind for a long time. We drove to the hospital and it seemed a very long drive. Chris was quite unaware of the significance of this journey, or that he was on his way to his last earthly home.

The staff in his ward were waiting for us and they gave him a very warm welcome.

His world had become very restricted and he loved their cheerful greetings and kind attention. His uncomplaining acceptance of this change made the path smoother for me, though I did find his unconcern for my needs or feelings hard. I often had to remind myself that his poor mind just could not cope. So I gave my sorrows to God.

On this day one year later I have written in my diary these words: 'On this day one year ago I stopped being the carer and became Chris's wife again.'

The relief was immense and now we were free to enjoy life a little. There were walks in the beautiful grounds and as I would push him around in his wheelchair I would sing to him. He used to love singing the old familiar hymns but now they were mostly gone from his mind and he could only join in little repetitive phrases. I sometimes think that I was singing to myself as much as to him.

Guide me Oh Thou Great Jehovah,
Pilgrim through this barren land,
I am weak but Thou art mighty,
Hold me with thy powerful hand.

The land seemed to be very barren now. I missed Chris and I felt alone. I certainly was weak, so asking God to hold me with his hand was no mere formality.

Things were good now in his new home, and mostly Chris was content. The nursing care was without fault so I could relax in confidence that he was being well cared for. There were lots of activities arranged in the hospital but as they were optional it meant that the patients and their families had choices. There was a lovely coffee shop that we often visited and there was also a little chapel near his ward. He loved the quietness and it seemed to calm his mind. The ministers visited from the church and a friend came regularly to read the Bible and pray with Chris, and this he seemed to enjoy.

But all was not always rosy. One day Terry pushed himself up to me in his wheelchair and shouted: 'Your husband is an IRA bastard. He was trying to get into my bed last night.'

'I think you might be mistaken,' I answered.

Terry was often vocal and angry. No way was he mistaken, he insisted. When I enquired of the nurse in charge, she said that indeed there had been a commotion the night before when Chris had propelled himself into Terry's space and tried to get into his empty bed.

I reasoned with Chris, 'You must not get into other people's beds.'

His answer surprised me. 'Oh yes,' he said, 'I go up and up till I find an empty bed and then I get into it.'

It set me thinking. There must have been a reason why he gave me this explanation. Chris's bed was halfway up the ward. He shared his little alcove with another man.

Light suddenly dawned on me. Chris didn't really know where his bed was and, as he needed a safe place of his own, he was finding 'home' the best way he knew how. I suggested this to the nurse in charge and she understood immediately.

'We must move him to a better place,' she said. 'Where would you like him to go? There are several free spots.' I could have hugged her!

We chose a corner at the end of the room beside a window, overlooking the lawn. In a flash they had moved Chris's bed and all his belongings. Now he had a cosy little 'home' that was to be his for the rest of his earthly life. So now both Chris and Terry were happy.

Other problems arose which were not so easily solved. It is said that spirituality and sexuality remain with the Alzheimer's sufferer after other characteristics have gone. This was true of Chris. His spirituality was a comfort to him, but his sexuality caused problems. As I wheeled him round the grounds of the hospital there were little alcoves and places where he would insist that, 'We stop here for a love,' and a 'love' didn't mean just a kiss! His persistence caused me quite a lot of distress and the more so because it was rather a private problem. Finally I had to tell the doctor who was in charge of Chris. She knew immediately what to do, and she prescribed a certain sedative that solved the problem. He was never doped but he was calm and we could enjoy our walks again.

Before Chris reached the end of his earthly journey, I suffered a small stroke and was admitted to the same hospital, where I was to remain for five weeks. The nurses pushed me down to his ward as soon as I was able. He was very matter of fact that I was ill and in a wheelchair. This was so unlike him and it made me sad.

As C.S. Lewis wrote, when his wife was terminally ill, 'We were setting out on different roads. "You, Madam to the right – you, Sir, to the left."'[1] Our bodies were meeting, each in our wheelchairs, but our hearts and minds were far apart.

I recovered well, but sadly Chris died of pneumonia on 2 January 2006. I lived through those days in a dream, and even as I write this account there is a sense of unreality and sorrow. Our children were a great support to me. I realise that it cannot have been easy for them to have both parents ill.

I am glad now that I was able to walk that grey road beside my husband in his time of need. As I remember many days of adversity I am thankful for those glimpses of glory which helped to brighten the way.

Note

[1]   C.S. Lewis (1966) *A Grief Observed.* London: Faber and Faber, p.14.

11

Our Mum Had To Be the Man of the House

The Malik family: Sania Malik and her daughters Ayesha, Aliyah and Fariha

As told to Lucy Whitman.

Sania: I came to England in 1984 when I got married. I was about nineteen and my husband was about 70. He had been living in England for a long time. He had been married before and his wife had died. He had two sons and a daughter from his first marriage. His daughter lives in Canada and we don't see her often but we have a close relationship with his sons.

I had three daughters with him. Ayesha is twenty and she is married now and goes out to work. Aliyah is seventeen and she is at college doing her A levels. Fariha is fourteen and she will soon be doing her GCSEs.

My husband started to become ill when we had been married about eight years. At first they said it was memory loss, then things started to get worse and they told us it was dementia.

Ayesha: He would do things like going out of the flat leaving the door open, turning on the gas without lighting it. There were times when he was out and about and he didn't know where he was. There was one time when the doctors actually thought he was mentally ill, so they put him in the mental hospital. From there they realised that he'd got dementia.

Sania: When Fariha was two and a half, I had a stroke and I had to go into hospital for two weeks. A social worker came and stayed to look after the children while I was in hospital, and when I came out they told me that my husband had to go into residential care. They could see that I couldn't manage to look after my children and my husband at the same time. They said it was too much for me, especially as I was ill myself. He was in a care home for four or five years, until they could no longer look after him and then he was in hospital for the next few years until he died, about eighteen months ago. By then he was in his nineties.

Ayesha: He went into the care home when I was about eight. I remember my dad before he became ill. He was a very hard worker. He was physically strong, because he used to do sports a lot, and wrestling, and all the manly things. I had a lot of fun with him. On my birthdays I miss him a lot, because I was so attached to him. He's gone now. I feel like I have lost a very close friend of mine.

Aliyah: I remember him taking us to nursery, but Fariha and I were too young to remember what he was really like.

Ayesha: But I do. I remember him very clearly. I know how he was before he got ill and I know how it went while he was ill, to the last stages. It was very distressing.

Aliyah: I was really young, and I don't think I realised too much that he was ill. Our mum brought us up. Now that I've grown older, in the past few years, I've realised how serious things were.

Ayesha: It was very different for me, compared to the others. I knew what was happening, and I saw my mum being ill at the same time as my father. It was like a heavy burden, when you're losing somebody that you're very attached to, and it really hurts.

Aliyah: She was the most upset, because she was older, and she was with Dad more. She cried a lot.

Sania: While he was in the care home he used to go once a week to the dementia care group at the day centre round the corner from where we live. And sometimes he would come and stay here for a few days.

Aliyah: The day centre was really good. We used to pop in to see him there. We used to enjoy going to see him. He used to recognise us sometimes, but there were times when he wouldn't remember us.

Ayesha: At the beginning it was okay, he would recognise us, but then he got worse. Sometimes he would get mixed up and he would think my mother was his daughter.

Sania: For me, the hardest thing was having young children to look after at the same time as looking after my husband. The care home and the hospital were quite far away and I had to take two buses to visit him. I went to see him about twice a week and I also had to attend so many appointments with the doctors and social workers and careworkers. It wasn't easy for me, going right across London, changing buses, and then coming back to get the children from school, doing the shopping and everything else.

My husband's brothers and sisters said to me, why was my husband in a care home?

Aliyah: They never took care of him. My mother took care of him. And then they used to blame my mother.

Sania: There was no choice! I said to my sister-in-law and brother-in-law, 'Take your brother, for one week you can look after him.'

Aliyah: The thing is, if we had been older, maybe we could have looked after ourselves, maybe our mum could have looked after him. But we were so young.

Ayesha: Their whole thinking was, 'It's all because of you,' as if our dad was ill because of our mum. 'You don't take care of him. You could take care of him at home if you liked!' No, she can't! It's not easy.

Aliyah: I don't think they saw a lot of how Dad's behaviour was. They hardly visited him at hospital. They didn't see how bad his situation was, what his behaviour was like. Even the doctors and the social workers were saying: 'You can't look after him.' Because my mum wasn't physically fit herself.

Ayesha: They knew my mum had been in hospital, but they just didn't accept it.

Sania: One day, he walked out of the care home and got on a bus and came back here to our flat. We weren't here. I had taken the girls to Pakistan for a holiday.

Aliyah: They were searching everywhere for him and in the end they found him sitting on the steps in our block of flats.

Ayesha: That was before he lost his mobility. He started to lose the ability to walk, and in the end he needed help to stand up. He got really worse in the last two or three years. He couldn't move much at all, he couldn't eat.

He also forgot how to speak. He used to speak English very well, but it disappeared completely. It just went. Then his Urdu started to go. In the home, they couldn't understand what he was saying. They would say, 'Can you translate for us?' But that was just for a couple of weeks, when he could just speak Urdu, and then that went as well. Everything was so sudden. One day he was speaking, and the next day, he's stopped speaking. It just got worse and worse.

I'm close to my mum, but I was closer to my dad. I've always opened out to him, from a very young age. I used to tell him everything. Whenever I was upset, I wouldn't tell my mum straight away, I used to go and speak to my dad first, even though he couldn't talk. I used to go and put my head on him, to calm myself down. Twice, I had a response from him, and it made me feel very calm afterwards. I was crying, and he just goes: 'Pray!'

Aliyah: He was a very holy man. He was very religious and he used to teach the Qur'an. Even when he couldn't speak much, he always used to say religious words. Sometimes, he would just come out with 'Allah!' Sometimes we would recite the Qur'an at his bedside or leave a tape of the Qur'an playing for him. He used to like listening to it.

Sania: When he was in the home, he sometimes touched the nurses in a sexual way, or he would suddenly drop his trousers.

Ayesha: Before his illness, he would never, ever do anything like that.

Aliyah: He was a holy man, very modest, and always respected women. We had to say sorry to the nurses, and tell them he was not really like that. Luckily, they understood that it was his illness and they didn't get angry with him.

Ayesha: When he finally died it was a big shock to me. I wasn't prepared for it. I had been told a few times that he didn't have long to live. I had kept on hearing them saying, 'Time is close, time is close,' but he always survived, so in the end I just thought, okay, nothing's going to happen to him. And then suddenly, one day, we got a phone call, saying he's passed away.

I was in a very bad state myself at the time. I was pregnant. I was coming on to my eighth month. I was quite ill and really weak. I was really stressed out by everything else, and the last thing I needed to know was that Dad had passed away. They were all trying to keep me calm.

After he died, I didn't really cry much, until after I had given birth, and then I broke down. I got the blues really badly after my baby was born.

Sania: After he had died, we quarrelled with my husband's family about where he was going to be buried.

Ayesha: We had a family gathering. It was the first time we had all met.

Aliyah: We had never met our half-sister, because she lives in Canada, but when our dad passed away, she came.

Ayesha: They were saying that my dad's grave should be in Pakistan. My mum said that she wants to send him there, but there was no one to actually go with him except for his brother, and he was being too stubborn.

Sania: My brother-in-law said, 'You take him!' I said, 'I can't take him – Ayesha's pregnant, she's not well, she's sick. You take him there.' He said, 'If you go, I'll go.' I said, 'Who will look after Ayesha?

Aliyah: In the end, he is buried here. He wanted to be buried in Pakistan, but we couldn't manage it. But if he was buried in Pakistan, we could hardly ever have visited. We could only go once in three years or so. Now he's buried here, we can go and see his grave.

Ayesha: My message to other people who have a family member who has dementia is: look after your elders, don't forget your loved ones. Even if they have to go into residential care, make sure you go and visit them.

Aliyah: We used to see some people in the home and in the hospital who didn't have any visitors. It's very sad.

Ayesha: Don't just forget about them. Show them you care.

Aliyah: I think what I have learned from this is that I need to work hard and get a good education so I can be independent. Our mum had to bring us up on her own.

Ayesha: She had to be the man of the house and the woman of the house. She had to be the father and mother at the same time. It was quite difficult for her.

Aliyah: She always worries about us more than anything else. She still wakes us up in the morning, 'Get ready for school, get ready for work.'

Ayesha: I am working now as a teaching assistant. I am helping children with special needs such as autism. I think that I have been affected by what happened to our family, to want to help others who need extra support.

Aliyah: My mum looks after Ayesha's daughter!

Ayesha: I've given her more work again!

Sania: I'm happy! With the small child, I'm happy.

Aliyah: Even when our dad passed away, the baby was one of the best things. It helped so much! It just changed everything and made us more happy!

12

On the Contrary

Lucy Whitman

My mother's descent into hell began when she fell and broke her leg, just below the hip, at the age of 88. The leg healed successfully, but something inside her stayed broken. The physiotherapist complained that she didn't seem very 'motivated' to get back on her feet again, as if she really ought to pull herself together.

While she was in hospital my father managed quite well on his own, although he himself had been seriously ill in recent years. But once my mum was back at home, he collapsed with one of the infections to which he was so susceptible. He was discovered lying on the bedroom floor, unable to get up, running a high temperature, insisting that he was perfectly well and forbidding all and sundry to call the doctor. My mother did not feel able to go against his wishes, but my sister and I overruled him when we found out what had happened. The doctor prescribed megastrength antibiotics, and we took it in turns to stay the night there until the fever and delirium subsided.

Still feeling fragile from her own fall, my mother was terrified by the fact that my father was ill and helpless as well. She no longer felt safe, and all her courage and confidence deserted her, never to return. She said it was 'as if a bomb had gone off' in her life. She had a commanding, resonant voice, which she had used to great effect in her years as a teacher, and at this stage she was still able to express herself forcefully, using vivid language.

My mother: Elizabeth Whitman, born 1910, survivor of two world wars and several family tragedies – most importantly, the death of her son, my brother Tony, killed in a car crash in 1967 at the age of 21. A loving mother and grandmother, a beloved aunt and great-aunt, she was also a lifelong pacifist, an outspoken campaigner against nuclear weapons. She had welcomed lodgers from all over the world into her home, and taught English as a second language for many years in adult education. Warm, hospitable and full of fun,

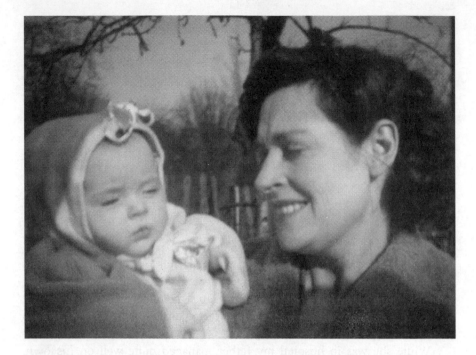

Elizabeth with Lucy as a baby

she loved giving parties, playing the piano and getting everyone to join in singing together.

This was the person we began to lose on that fateful day of her first fall. Of course, we did not know this at the time. After this fall, there was a period of nearly two years during which she declined, not at a steady pace, but in fits and starts.

Like my father, she became subject to repeated urinary tract infections (UTIs) which, in medical parlance, made her 'confused'. This seemed like an understatement to us, as she was in some instances literally raving – but at this stage she always more or less returned to 'normal' after these distressing interludes. When she was in the grip of these infections, she became extremely suspicious of everyone about her, telling me in no uncertain terms that the hospital nurses were 'only in it for the money', and accusing my sister and me of treating her with heartless cruelty when we tried to arrange for her to go into respite care. She raged at us like King Lear berating his ungrateful daughters Goneril and Regan:

> *Lear.* How sharper than a serpent's tooth it is
> To have a thankless child![1]

Lear. ...you unnatural hags,
> I will have such revenges on you both
> That all the world shall – I will do such things,
> What they are, yet I know not, but they shall be
> The terrors of the earth...[2]

She had several spells in hospital as a result of these UTIs, and during these episodes, she frequently antagonised the staff, accusing them of treating her rudely and unkindly. We felt embarrassed by the scenes she was making, and tried to smooth things over. At the time, we were still trying to reason with her and get her to behave 'sensibly' and in her own best interests. We didn't realise that she had passed into a land beyond reason, and beyond normal social skills – a land of pure emotion where she was suffering and everyone else was to blame.

With hindsight, I now feel very disappointed that the hospital staff were so ill-prepared to meet the needs of their aged patients, many of whom clearly had dementia. They responded to her constant demands for attention and accusations of neglect as one would to a perfectly rational person who was choosing to be obnoxious – a 'cantankerous old woman' – seemingly oblivious to the fact that her behaviour was a symptom of her illness rather than an unpleasant flaw in her personality.

In addition to the UTIs, it is now clear that our mother also suffered a number of 'mini-strokes', each of which left her mind and body feebler than the last. We were not really aware that these were happening at the time, but on one occasion my sister Rosalind visited and found that one side of Mum's face was numb. She could not speak coherently, and when she tried to play the piano, all she could produce was a strange cacophony.

'But you can hear the music that's inside my head, can't you dear?' she said, to my sister's consternation.

Both my parents were great readers, and particularly loved nineteenth-century novelists such as Dickens. My father had been registered partially sighted by this time, but he arranged for the mobile library to visit the house, bringing a selection of large-print books which he hoped my mother would find comforting. Unfortunately, it became obvious that my mother could no longer make sense of the printed word – especially the long and complicated sentences beloved of the Victorians. One sad day, my mother struggled to make head or tail of the opening paragraph of one of Thomas Hardy's novels. It was a book she had read and enjoyed in the past, but now the convoluted syntax defeated her. 'I must be getting silly,' she said forlornly, and my father tried to come to the rescue. I witnessed a poignant scene, as my father – who had macular degeneration, meaning that he could only see one or two words

at a time, if he squinted out of the corner of his eye, through a powerful mag-
nifying glass – tried to see enough of the sentence to help my mother make
sense of it, when she could not hold in her mind the words he had managed
to identify a few seconds before. Between them they could not get hold of
enough words at once to make any sense of the text.

My mother became very depressed. She was terrified of having another
fall, and became more and more reluctant to walk about at all, even to shuffle
from one room to another with the help of her walking frame. We borrowed
a wheelchair to take her out, but she hated the sensation of being wheeled
around, and seemed to expect to be tipped out at any moment. A doctor upset
her enormously by telling her that an x-ray had shown that her spine was
'crumbling badly' with osteoporosis. Worst of all, she was painfully aware
that her mental faculties were deserting her – as if her brain, as well as her
spine, were crumbling away, and there was nothing she could do about it.

My sister and I both visited several times a week, but it was never enough.
You could go round, spend three or four hours there, get home, and as you
walked in the door, the phone would ring:

'When are you coming to see me? I would have thought you could have
made a bit more effort...'

Then she had another fall. This time it was as if she had toppled right
over a cliff. She clung on to the edge for a few days, but soon lost her grip
completely and slithered down the precipice into the abyss.

I kept her company in the accident and emergency ward that evening,
while she waited to be examined. Despite the shock of the fall, she was in
good form. Although she was quite unable to give the right answers to the
questions which are used to assess mental functioning, she was not in pain,
and we had quite a jolly and companionable time. This was the last evening
my mother and I spent together, when she was truly herself, and truly knew
who I was.

My sister and I both went to see her every day. Each time we visited, she
was vaguer and more confused than the last.

'Oh it's lovely to see you, dear,' she told me after a few days, 'but you can
only come once a week, can't you?'

'Mum!' I protested, 'I've been coming every day!'

If I arrived at 4 o'clock, aware that someone else had been there until 3,
she would tell me she had not had any visitors all day.

'And what do you think about this idea they've got, of trying to get me
to have another baby?' she suddenly exclaimed.

My sister had the idea of trying to help her stay alert by doing some
'mental exercises'. She asked her a series of questions about the family, including all our names, and to her dismay, found she couldn't answer any of them.

When she asked, 'What is your husband's name?' Mum thought hard for a long time and eventually said, 'John'. When my sister said gently, 'No, it's not John, it's George, and you know that, because you are always calling out for him,' Mum replied scornfully, 'Yes, but that's not his *real* name, that's just what *I* call him.' Mum lay back on her pillow and rounded off the conversation by saying, 'Well, you must be very tired now, because you're not well, so I shall go now.'

There was no medical need for her to stay in hospital very long, but social services were slow to organise the follow-up care without which she could not be discharged. She ended up staying in hospital for five weeks, and during that time her condition deteriorated beyond repair. She lost the ability to answer even the simplest question, such as 'Are you feeling tired?' Finishing a sentence, completing a thought, became too much for her. 'On the contrary...' she said emphatically, several times, as she tried to pin down the ideas floating about in her mind. We never did find out what she was referring to. But she knew that something was seriously amiss, and needed to be put right.

What amazes me, in retrospect, is that the nurses and doctors were seemingly oblivious to the terrible drama which was unfolding before their eyes. We tried to talk to them, to say, 'Our mother is getting worse, not better... She's not usually like this... We're afraid that we are losing her completely...' We drew a blank. The only response we got was the usual explanation that she was a bit 'confused', as if there wasn't much to worry about. So long as they were monitoring her blood pressure and her temperature, giving her the prescribed medication and making sure she didn't fall over again, they felt their job was done.

Not one person acknowledged that our mother had suddenly plunged into an advanced state of dementia, not one person sat us down and talked to us about what this might mean for our mother and for the rest of the family. Not one person gave us any recognition of the fact that all of a sudden, our mother had been taken from us, as surely as if she had died in her hospital bed. Why was there so little explicit recognition of dementia, in a care of the elderly ward, of all places?

We were concerned that the longer she stayed in hospital, the more damage was being done to her brain, and the less likelihood there was that she would ever recover her wits – but what we had to say was of no interest to the ward staff. It did not seem to occur to them that a sudden steep deterioration in mental function should be taken just as seriously as any marked physical change. Even if there was nothing they could do about it, they should have been prepared to talk to us about what was going on. We needed a diagnosis of our mother's condition, and we certainly needed support both in coming to terms with it and planning how we could best look after her in this new situation.

The social workers seemed equally determined to ignore what we told them. Just before my mother was discharged, I spoke on the phone to the team which arranges care for frail elderly patients when they get home from hospital. They told me they would be interviewing my mother to assess her needs. I spent a long time explaining to them in graphic detail how my mother was now unable to speak coherently, that she was uncertain of where she was, and not in any fit state to tell them what she needed in terms of daily care. I requested what I thought would be an appropriate level of care on her behalf. However, protocol required that they should still meet her personally to assess her themselves. Fair enough. Except that I then received another call from the social worker, telling me in an exasperated way that she had not been able to get any sense out of my mother, to find out what her needs were, because 'she's completely demented!' Throughout her long stay in hospital, the word dementia had never once been uttered by the nurses or doctors, even in response to all the concerns we had expressed. For it to be mentioned in this brutally casual way was like being stabbed in the heart.

We had held out a faint hope that once she was back in familiar surroundings, she would become more like her old self, but no such luck. She did not even recognise her home when she got there, and almost immediately forgot all about her long stay in hospital. We had to accept that she would not recover.

Some people with dementia do not appear to be unhappy. Sadly, this was not the case with our mother. For the last few months of her life, she suffered excruciating grief and terror. She was trapped in a hell as agonising as anything the medieval theologians could have envisaged. She could not bear to be left alone even for a second. 'Frightened!' she kept on saying, 'Terrified!'

She could not usually explain what she was frightened about, but once when I asked her, she said, 'Because I can't do anything.' She was horribly aware that she was losing her grip. 'I am going funny in the head, you know,' she said to my sister.

Nothing we could do or say could comfort her or ease her torment. She didn't want to listen to the radio, and wouldn't let us read to her, saying, 'No, no, I don't understand.'

One of the most painful things, for me, was that she could no longer bear to hear me sing. She had encouraged me to sing since my earliest childhood, and had always taken pleasure in my voice. Now when I tried singing gently to her to try to soothe her, she begged me to stop. 'No! No! No!' she moaned, as if I were scraping my fingernails down a blackboard.

I tried talking to her about the family, the old days, but she couldn't bear that either. The past had always been very important to her, very vivid in her mind, and all my life she had enjoyed talking about her mother, and what things had been like years ago.

'Do you remember when I was a little girl...' I began.

'Why? What about it?' she interrupted fiercely, so that it was impossible for me to go on. I think she must have been afraid that she would *not* remember, and didn't want to be caught out.

I thought that maybe it would help if she could talk about death, and what she expected to find.

'What do you think it will be like?' I asked. 'Do you think you will see your loved ones again, like Tony?'

She looked very puzzled. 'I don't remember...'

It was terrible to discover that she no longer remembered that she had had a son who had died – probably the most deeply felt experience of her life.

The one person who she did remember clearly, and longed for, was her 'dear Mother', who had died in 1942.

'Is it true', she said incredulously, 'that my mother isn't here?'

Calling out for my father became a habit, a sort of automatic reflex, but soon his name became distorted. 'George! George!' turned into 'Joe! Joe!' and even, sometimes, 'Jones!' or 'Joge!' or 'Jorks!'

Above all, our mother longed for rest.

Mother: I want to go home.

Lucy: But Mum, you *are* at home.

Mother: I want to go to bed.

Lucy: But Mum, you *are* in bed.

Mother: Want *more* bed.

Our dad amazed us by the way he rose to the challenge of supporting her through this final stage in her illness. For the rest of us, an hour or two in her company was as much as we could bear, with the endless bleating for the non-existent Joe, but he stayed with her day and night, except for the interludes when we gave him a break. He had always cherished solitude, and had spent most of his married life cloistered in his study working or reading, yet he stayed by her side, infinitely kind and patient, never showing the least sign of irritation or desperation.

It took a long time to accept that my mother was never going to get any better – indeed, that she could only get worse – and it was only gradually

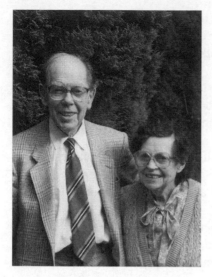

George and Elizabeth

that I recognised that what was tearing me apart was not just anxiety or stress or exhaustion, as I had thought, but grief.

My sister and I were run off our feet with everything we had to do to make sure our mother was all right, taking our dad to his numerous hospital appointments, managing their money affairs, arranging urgent repairs to their rambling old house – and all this on top of all our own work and family responsibilities. My friends and colleagues knew I was under a strain, and made kindly enquiries from time to time, but nobody realised – not even me – that actually I was suffering the agonies of grief: I was in mourning, because we had already lost her.

After some delay, we managed to get her assessed by the community mental health consultant, who confirmed that she was suffering from vascular dementia. The actual diagnosis brought us some help – but of course by this stage her dementia was at an advanced stage, and her condition was deteriorating with alarming speed.

When the consultant visited, my mother was sitting up in bed. My sister and I were both present, and Mum's carer also happened to be in the room, sorting out some laundry.

'Can you tell me who all these people are?' the consultant asked.

'Well, I was just going to ask you that,' replied my mum. After giving the matter some thought, she decided that we were her sisters – not a bad guess, really.

Although she was not quite sure who we were, and certainly could not name us any longer, she still seemed to recognise us at some level as people who were important to her and cared about her. When I visited on my own, she often asked me about 'the boy', meaning my son, so she still knew that I was the one who had a boy. Although it felt as though nothing we could do could ease her suffering, I am convinced that Dad's constant presence, and our frequent visits, did make a difference.

My mother's appetite had been poor for some time. Now it became difficult to get her to eat anything at all. She got thinner and thinner. I was shocked one day to see her without her clothes. Her breasts – which long ago had suckled me – had vanished completely.

It was not so long ago that I had watched with pleasure as my son learnt to eat solid food, and walk, and talk, and go to the toilet on his own. Now I had a grim 'running the film backwards' experience, as my mother progressively forgot how to do all these things.

When we were children she had taught us to say our prayers, to believe in a loving God who would take care of us. I had long since ceased to be a believer, but it saddened me to find that religion was of absolutely no use to her as she faced her own death and dissolution. She had completely forgotten about the very idea of God the Father. Only her Dear Mother mattered to her now.

My mother's illness made me wonder about the very nature of human identity. Where did our mother go, when she lost her wits? All her memories, her thoughts, her beliefs, almost everything which made her herself, seemed to have been erased. It was as if she had not only forgotten who *we* were, she had forgotten who *she* was. Was she still in there somewhere, out of reach of herself and us?

The day before she died, I lay on the bed with her, holding her hand.

'I'm Lucy, I'm your daughter, and I love you,' I said, over and over again. She could hardly speak. Another stroke had half paralysed her mouth. But I thought I heard her say, 'Love daughter.'

The next day, my sister and I spent the afternoon and evening at her side with Dad.

'We're all here,' we told her, 'George and Rosalind and Lucy. We are your family. We are with you and we love you…'

She could hardly move her mouth, but she said something which sounded like, 'You too.'

When night came, Dad went to sleep on the bed next to her, and my sister and I took it in turns to stay awake. She was sinking further and further into unconsciousness. A big sigh suddenly rippled through her, and we watched, as the last traces of our mother gradually left her body. The latest stroke had left her twisted and drooping, and her head had fallen so much to one side that it almost looked as if it were fixed on upside down. She looked like a tiny baby bird that had fallen out of its nest. And yet she looked comfortable, at last.

We stayed up all night. At dawn we looked out of the window to see the huge yew tree outside lit up, completely transfigured by the rising sun, radiant as an angel.

Some members of the choir I sing with, which my mother had also belonged to, came and sang at her funeral. One of the songs they sang was the spiritual, 'By and by', a joyous-sounding air, holding out the promise of rest for the weary and troubled:

Oh by and by, by and by,
I'm going to lay down my heavy load...

It is the words of the verse which lay bare the suffering behind this longing:

I know my robe's going to fit me well
(I'm going to lay down my heavy load)
I tried it on at the gates of hell
(I'm going to lay down my heavy load)[3]

At last my mother had been released from her hell. At last she was at peace.

Notes

[1] Shakespeare, *King Lear*, Act 1, Scene 4.
[2] Shakespeare, *King Lear*, Act 2, Scene 4.
[3] Traditional spiritual, arranged by Michael Tippett for his oratorio, *A Child of Our Time*. Tippett, M. (1944) *A Child of Our Time*. London: Schott and Co., pp.74–76.

13

*F*amily Matters

Ian McQueen

The poet John Donne was right about no man being an island. Illness affects not just the patient, but also his or her partner, children, family and friends. This was certainly true in my own family and also in that of my parents' oldest friends.

My mother Liz was born in 1926, 'the same year as the Queen!' as she often remarked. My father John was seven years older, and they both came from the same Lanarkshire mining village, long since subsumed into the Glasgow conurbation. They were married in the early 1950s, and Liz moved to London where John was then working. By the time they returned in 1959, I – their only son – had been born. Scotland was where I spent my formative years. I returned to London to study in the early seventies, and never moved back to Glasgow.

Dad did well in the civil service, right up to the 1970s. When given promotion to an Edinburgh office, he commuted back and forth from Glasgow, rather than move house. This was so as not to disturb me during my O level studies. That's the kind of dedicated husband and father my dad was. Then Dad's mother became forgetful, and started to repeat herself constantly: she'd 'gone senile'.

Dad's sister suggested their mother move close beside her, then promptly ignored her. After she began to wander at night (in search of her home years before in Edinburgh) her children decided that they would take turns looking after her. John had her for six months, then he and Liz went on holiday while his mum went to his sister's. On their return, however, he found that his mother was in a large asylum, about twenty miles away, in north Lanarkshire.

My grandmother had been found in the street at 1 o'clock in the morning, shouting: 'This isnae ma hoose! Ah wahnt tae go back tae ma ain hoose!' So

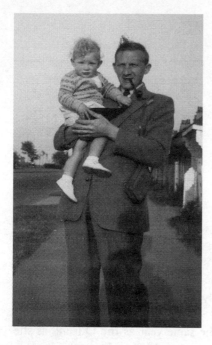

Ian with his father John, c.1958

there was no way they could continue to look after her then, of course.

Dad was upset, but there seemed no alternative.

The asylum was a huge barn of a place – a cross between a stately home in the highlands and a Victorian prison. Wards were locked and the residents were referred to as 'Granny' by staff. Their clothes were not the clothes they'd brought with them, and they sat in a pale thin line opposite each other, along the wall under the tall windows, until they were visited or led off to a meal. My gran and I wept together when I first visited her. A couple of years later, in 1973, she died. She was 84. At my last visit she hadn't known me. Soon, it was all forgotten, or rather, we tried to forget.

My mother Liz was a gregarious woman but her lack of confidence was made worse by John's insistence on taking care of all bills and financial decision-making. He'd discouraged her from taking a civil service examination or from learning to drive. In some ways, then, John was a typical 'I'm in charge' man of his generation. But in other ways, thank goodness, he was quite different! He was a bookish, quiet, self-sufficient type. He'd joined an English regiment in 1939, and had served and been decorated at Alamein and Monte Cassino. To John, family was everything. My mother and I were his *raison d'être*.

By 1980, my father was a manager in a large office to the south-east of Glasgow. But he was feeling the strain. There were 60 members of staff – no wonder he forgot their names! 'Then give it up,' urged Mum, obviously saying what her husband wanted to hear. 'You're more important than the money.'

So he retired at 60 to his garden, endless summers of golf and occasional trips south to visit me in London. This continued for twenty years.

In 2001, I organised a golden wedding celebration for my parents on Lanzarote. Things went well at first, but a few days before we were to return home, Dad became ill with bowel problems and had to have a minor operation. It was a severe blow to his confidence. He was no longer, it seemed, 'in charge'.

The following summer, he began to forget people's names when he and Liz bumped into them on the street or in the supermarket. He was very adept at covering it up at first: 'Oh, don't be silly!' he'd look askance at Liz. 'Of course I know who they are!' But he still didn't say their names.

Gradually, he became depressed. He was insecure about money. ('Are you sure we can afford that?') He kept cutting the shrubs in the borders down to the ground, manically. He'd visit his sisters and start fingering all their knick-knacks and gadgets, like a small boy with his toys. When I brought my old friend Paul to visit my parents, and Paul left the room for a minute, Dad effusively greeted him on his return, as if he'd just turned up!

This kind of thing got to be a severe strain on Liz. She worried and she lost weight. Then there were nightmares. Dad would writhe across the bed in his sleep, moaning and re-living the terrible wartime experiences he'd kept bottled up all these years. Their next-door neighbour had to come in one night and call for an ambulance. The paramedics were kind, and calmed John down, but Liz became more and more tired. Would I come up to stay, and let her go on holiday with her cousin to the Isle of Wight?

The week was glorious: long days of endless sunshine. Dad and I went to visit his old chums at the golf club, but he couldn't put a name to them. In the evening, we listened to the Proms together, on the radio. But, at night, there were the same nightmares. Once, Dad called out to know where his parents

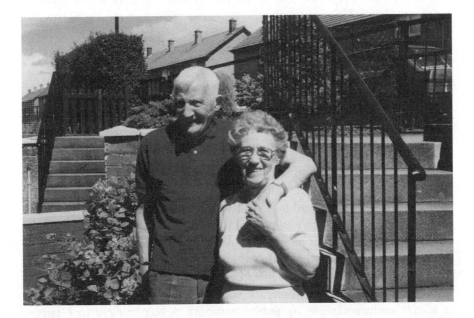

John and Liz, 1996

were. When I explained that he was 82 years old and that, sadly, his parents were dead, he burst into paroxysms of grief and begged to be taken to visit their graves. NHS Direct could offer no counsel. The GP prescribed more anti-depressants. Dad told me he was unsure of how to get back home if he went for a walk. He told a fellow swimmer at the local pool, jokingly, that he'd no idea where his locker was. But I was listening and watching: 'Don't worry, Dad, I know where it is!' Clearly, something would have to be done on Mum's return.

The GP had another idea: a mental health assessment programme at the local day hospital. John went for an initial interview. He was asked who the prime minister of the day was and how to spell 'world' backwards. He managed the latter. He then started going to a pleasant day centre twice a week. The front door bell rang and John happily committed himself into the hands of two young women who took him to the minibus and returned him at 4.30. He never spoke about what had happened at the hospital, but he obviously enjoyed himself at the day centre, where he could practise his golf, and Liz enjoyed some blissful respite.

John became more withdrawn, and started lying in bed later and later each day. Liz was becoming exhausted as she traipsed up and down stairs with trays. She lost more weight. The gerontologist advised Mum and me to visit nursing homes. 'I'm not saying for now,' he ventured sagely. 'You'll know when...' I drove her round four or five homes in the vicinity. One smelled of urine. One had two separate regimes: upstairs were the physically boisterous, even aggressive residents. Doors to the outside were locked. Downstairs, a more easygoing attitude prevailed. But neither Mum nor I could forget the cries from above.

Shortly after this, my father was diagnosed with Alzheimer's.

At Christmas 2003, I went up to Glasgow. I was accosted in my parents' road by a neighbour. 'Can't you see what this is doing to your mother? When are you going to do something?'

I looked at my mother in a new light. She'd lost nearly two and a half stones. I was precipitated into action and, as soon as the new year celebrations were over, Dad went into the nursing home for a trial period of one month's 'respite'. For both Mum and myself, it felt like a major betrayal. How could we leave him there and drive away? But there seemed no alternative, given the effect of the previous four months on my mother, and our apprehension as to what might follow. Now, Liz weighed in at just six and a half stones.

It was the home Mum had liked best. It wasn't a local authority institution but a private nursing home, for which a 'top-up' fee was payable. And it wasn't easily accessible by public transport. A bus halfway to Glasgow city centre in one direction had to be followed by another bus back again in another direction. And being a canny Scot, Liz decided, yes, she'd get a taxi there but she'd walk back a mile or so in order to catch only one bus home.

John settled in. After the initial trial period, I came back for a meeting with Mum, Dad, the administrator of the home and the social worker. Dad was articulate during the proceedings. He didn't want to be separated from his family, he said, but if contact could be maintained, he didn't mind staying there. Mum cried herself to sleep that night.

And so, some sort of routine began. Every day, Saturday and Sunday included, my mother made the journey to see my father. The care staff was very variable. There was one Irish staff nurse who took a special interest in Dad, but many of the 'carers' were quite uncaring. He could still charm the women: 'It's a pleasure tae help John, he's a real gent!' Liz felt torn, even guilty, at leaving him each time; she'd think of the 50 odd years they'd spent together, as he stood framed in the lounge window, waving to her, while she stood alone in the car park. And gradually, inexorably, John's Alzheimer's got worse. He became more and more helpless – closing his mind, it seemed, to this demeaning situation.

The home wasn't too unpleasant. It was just institutional and impersonal. Everything was subject to shifts, routines and procedures. Nothing was human, in the sense of being individually tailored to helping each resident grow and develop as a human being. It was all about feeding the body, keeping it clean, and pretending the mind or spirit was somebody else's concern. Oh, there were some very dedicated nurses and a pleasant administrator, and the owner arranged a visit one day to her hotel on the coast. There was also a social organiser who arranged for a musician to come in and lead a sing-song occasionally, on residents' birthdays. But Dad got out very little.

Some items of his, like an expensive shaver Liz had given him for a birthday present, went missing and he often wore clothes which weren't his. Liz seethed! He had bumps and bruises which couldn't be explained. Then, late in the summer, he began to try opening the emergency exits to try to get out. Finally, he fell and sustained serious cuts and bruises, trying to get down the internal fire escape from the room he shared on the first floor.

At last, he escaped and made his way round the corner (of the main road outside!) into a little adjacent housing estate, and into someone's house. Luckily, the owner was one of the care staff who knew him and returned him to the home.

Liz naturally became more and more worried, and more and more exhausted. I went up sometimes, by car from London, and drove my mother and father to the local loch they'd often enjoyed walking round, or to a garden centre on the tourist route down the Clyde Valley. Liz also went to

London for a break now and again. But every day she phoned the nursing home, and every day she was away she felt guilty.

Early in 2005, John stopped talking. He sometimes uttered a few intelligible words, but then he drifted into apparent gibberish and silence. He was now doubly incontinent. Liz took him offerings of sweets and drinks which he ate while she carried on a kind of monologue to which John paid increasingly little heed.

By this time, the focus of my attention and concerns had moved from father to mother, as Liz became weaker. She could no longer walk the mile uphill between one bus route and another. The visits became shorter and Dad's ability to engage and respond to her lessened. More often than not, when he had a visitor, he seemed to be asleep. Liz became convinced that it was the drugs he was taking which were designed to keep him subdued. A member of the gerontology team conducted some experiments to check John's voluntary and involuntary response to external stimuli like voices or physical gestures. He concluded that John was *not* being controlled by sedation. His brain was somehow *rejecting* these stimuli and *choosing* to ignore them. The anti-depressant medication had been previously adjusted after the aggressive phase. Aricept had also been temporarily administered in the hope it could arrest or temporarily halt the progress of John's Alzheimer's. If it did help at all, its effect was negligible.

In February 2006, my mother suffered a heart attack. She was hospitalised and, for a time, I had to take time off and visit both parents in different institutions in different parts of Glasgow. A few weeks later, Dad became unable to eat or drink, but apparently this was not grounds for his admission to hospital. Only when he began to bleed from his rectum was he finally admitted. And now began a kind of cat-and-mouse game between life and death. 'He may recover,' the doctors said. ('But he can't eat or drink!') 'He could go to a long-term stay hospital,' the doctors said. ('But he can't open his eyes.') What was my father's quality of life at this time? His body was quietly, scarcely noticeably, registering its protest that his quality of life was nil.

My mother and I watched him; moistened his lips with a kind of red lollipop thing and waited for the inevitable. When it came, it was like a blessed relief. Dad was 86.

Coincidentally, while all this was going on, my mother's best friend Janet had also begun to show signs of dementia. My mother had known Janet ever since they were girls, and despite various ups and downs over the years, their friendship survived into old age.

Janet's husband William had been shaped by his working class upbringing. He was a joiner on Clydeside – apparently he'd built the QEII almost single-handedly! In 2001, he succumbed to the asbestos exposure he'd experienced at work, years before, and died of cancer after a sadly short retirement.

Janet never really recovered. She gradually deteriorated, complaining that she couldn't cope on her own. Her younger son, Rob, had to reduce his hours as a university lecturer to look after her. He had recently retrained as a minister of the Church of Scotland, but he deferred applying for a post in the ministry as he felt he had to be there for his mother.

Rob's caring regime was strict. He didn't allow the TV on in the evenings, nor the nightly tipple of whisky (heavily diluted with Irn-Bru) which Janet and William had once enjoyed. Janet became more and more inward-looking. She complained constantly of aches and pains. She was very prone to cystitis, it seemed, and Rob was often heard to cajole her: 'Drink your tea, mother.'

Once, my mother received a call from a couple who were living in the house where Janet's late mother used to live. Apparently, Janet had walked the half-mile or so from her own house to bang on their door and demand: 'Where's mah mammy?!' The couple had found Liz's name in Janet's purse. And so Liz went round and sat with Janet until her granddaughter arrived to take Janet home. I rang up Janet's elder son, Craig, to plead with him that my mother had enough to worry about without being concerned about looking after Janet!

Eventually, in late 2007, the two brothers found Janet a place in a Christian nursing home in a lovely setting in south Lanarkshire. Janet settled in well: it was more like a hotel. And yet, it was twenty miles away from their home town and they only saw their mother once a week.

Janet died in early 2008. Liz was very happy to have seen her friend, briefly, one last time a few weeks before, but found she was very confused. 'You're not Liz,' was all she'd said.

Janet's son Rob couldn't bear to attend the funeral. Shortly afterwards, he became a voluntary patient in a Glasgow mental hospital. He had discovered that by giving up full-time work to look after Janet, he'd missed a five-year deadline, after which he could no longer apply for jobs in the ministry, under Church of Scotland rules. It was not the kind of thing newly ordained clergy should forget. But, perhaps, in the circumstances, it was not surprising that he had.

After all this sadness, my mother Liz has started to lead a strange new life as a homeowner and member of the church guild. At first she felt, having lost both husband and best friend, that her role – her place in the community – had been usurped, but now she is beginning to make new friends.

I asked her to move to London, but at the age of 82, she is beginning to enjoy her new-found independence. If a granny flat or a bigger house were a possibility in London, then she might consider it, but in the meantime, there are her lovely neighbours. She can afford a gardener to complain about. And those lovely nieces who visit when they can, and the holidays to France and Italy with me are great, so long as her health is up to it...

Yes, all in all, she is doing all right.[1]

Note

[1]   Some names have been changed.

14

Back and Forth

Geraldine McCarthy

As told to Lucy Whitman.

The first time I became aware of my father not being himself was about 1995. I took my dad and mum away to West Cork for the weekend. They rarely got to go away. They never had a car. Holidays weren't something we did as kids. So for them to get away like this was quite an unusual thing. On the Friday night we had dinner and played cards together, and then went off to bed. The room that my mum and dad slept in was on the ground floor, and I was sleeping above them in this kind of half-open attic space. I was upstairs in bed, and I could hear my mum and dad below. And I heard my father saying to my mother, 'Clare, are they all home? Is the back door locked?'

And Mum went, 'Jack, what are you saying? We're away with Geraldine.'

And then there was a bit of a pause, and then he said again, 'Are all the children home, Clare?'

And I was upstairs thinking this was very odd! All six of us had grown up long ago. I never said anything to my mum or dad the next day, partly because I felt I was intruding on their privacy, because of the layout of the house. So I felt a bit awkward, but it stuck in my mind. There were a few other moments which were a bit puzzling, but I didn't really think any more about it.

I moved to London in 1997, and about a year or so later Dad had a fall. He used to cycle everywhere. He was a cyclist when he was younger. He used to cycle races and win cups, and he was still cycling at this point, when he was in his eighties. But this particular day when he went out he fell off his bike – fortunately, just at the front gate. It did something to his hip, and he ended up in the orthopaedic hospital. That fall aged him. It marked the beginning of a deterioration that people couldn't ignore. It speeded something up.

Dad was a mason by trade. He had these really solid builder's hands: there was a real strength to them, and a real gentleness. And in a way that's what he was like. He was quite a stern man when he wanted to be, quite set in his ways, quite traditional and conservative. And then there was a real gentleness about him, and a real 'devilment' as well. One of the things people would always say about my father was that he had this twinkle in his eye. And the other part of him – the quite stubborn part of him – was sometimes challenging, especially as he got older, because he wouldn't let anybody else do things. He was the man who looked after the house: if the house needed painting, if something needed done in the house, he did it. If he couldn't do it, he found it very hard to think about anybody else doing it, which used to make life a bit of a struggle for my mum, I think. When he was in his seventies and eighties, we'd come home to find him up on the roof, cleaning out the gutters or something! But he just thought, 'Have ladder, will go on roof…' There was something in him you just couldn't get around. I remember trying to negotiate with him to go and get his ears tested for a hearing aid. No, no, no. Absolutely no way.

My father absolutely adored my mother. He loved her to bits. And she him as well. I can remember when I was small, they would sometimes go to a dinner dance at Christmas. And when Mammy would come out of the bedroom, when she'd be dressed, my father would say, 'Look at your mother, now. Isn't she beautiful?' There was always that sense that he was extremely proud of her. But that element of his personality which went 'No!' – that probably led to some struggles in their relationship, particularly when they were first married. But the front that they presented to us was always very united. And at home, in the sitting room, there were two armchairs on either side of the fire, and my father sat in one and my mother sat in the other.

Since Dad had retired, they had a very quiet existence. They were very, very close as a couple. I think that was an advantage, but it made it harder when Dad's dementia developed. His illness really restricted my mother. There was a period of time when he would follow her everywhere. If she got up to go to the kitchen, to go to the bathroom, he would be behind her. So she started to just sit, a lot of the time, to keep him safe. Putting it bluntly, her life just became sitting at home so that my father would not be alone.

I sometimes felt as if my brothers and sisters judged my mum, as if she had stopped trying, especially because as the years went on, it was starting to affect her own mobility and abilities. I think there was a feeling that she should get up and try and do more. They would say, 'She could have gone out, she could have done things if she'd wanted to.' And I remember saying, 'But we can't know what she's feeling. He's our dad, but he's her *husband*. He's her life partner of 60 years.'

The last four or five years of his illness were the hardest, but I think that the earlier years were probably very challenging for my mother too. I suspect she kept a lot from us, and that we only heard and saw the tip of the iceberg.

She was the one spending most of her time with him. For the first few years, there weren't carers coming into the house. He was still able to eat and take himself to the loo and do all of those things, so the care was being done by the family, primarily my mother. And when you'd visit, you'd be sitting talking, and she would find different ways of including him in the conversation, if she felt he wasn't following it. But sometimes you'd notice that if she was feeling tired or a bit stressed, she just found it too hard, the effort and the energy it took, and she'd get kind of agitated. Sometimes she would just want to sit and have a conversation. She was with him 24/7. What we would experience, visiting for a few hours, she was having all of the time.

After his fall, my dad got an amazing amount of mobility back. He had this very particular way of walking, because the hip never quite straightened fully again, but he could get about, and he could pick up speed when he wanted to! My parents' house is now on the suburbs of Cork city, but when I was growing up it was pure country. When you come outside my mum and dad's door, there's just fields, but all you have to do is walk three minutes, and you're on to a main road. My dad still wanted to ride his bike, but Mum decided, after a few hairy episodes, that the bike needed to be locked, and the key put somewhere that he wouldn't find it. And for a long time that was fine. But one day he spent hours, back and forth, back and forth, looking for the key for the bike, in all these different places. And he found another key, that my mum didn't know about, and he unlocked the bike and tried to take it out again! And after that the bike had to be 'disappeared' completely.

My father used to get very anxious. He'd go from being quite relaxed to suddenly getting agitated and thinking he had to go somewhere, or there was something he had to do. 'Will we go home now? Is it time to go home?'

And we'd say, 'Dad, you're all right, you're at home, you don't have to go anywhere, you're grand.'

And he'd go, 'Oh, right, right, right.' And he'd sit down. But it took a while before he relaxed again.

There was one day when he thought he wasn't at home, and I said, 'You *are* at home, Dad. This is your house.'

And he went, 'Oh? Is it?'

And I said, 'Yes, it is. It's a grand house, isn't it?'

'Have I been here long?'

'Yes, you've lived here a long time, 60 or more years.'

And I was telling him stuff about the house, and he said, 'You seem to know this place very well.'

And I said, 'That's because I lived here, too.'

'Did you?'

'Yes, I lived here for eighteen years.'

'Did you?'

'Yes. And guess what!'

'What?'

'I'm your daughter.'

And he went, '*Are* you? Pleased to meet you!' and he shook my hand.

And the way he went, 'Pleased to meet you' – that *was* my father. When you brought someone to the house, and said, 'Dad, this is so-and-so,' he'd go, 'Pleased to meet you!' and he'd stand up and shake their hand.

Another time, I was just sitting there, making conversation. And I looked up, and he was making this sweeping movement with his hands, and I said, 'What are you doing, Dad?' and he said, 'Getting the cows home.' My father's father was a farm labourer, so when my father was a little child in the 1920s, he would have sometimes gone with my grandfather to different farms. So he was getting the cows home...

When I left Ireland, I was a grown woman. I made a conscious decision to move away from my family to come here to England to be with my partner, Helen. It was very hard, because I knew I was moving away from my parents who were already ageing. When it became apparent that my father had dementia, it put an additional strain on me, because I felt far away.

When you're the person who's not there all the time, your brothers and sisters who are there every day are dealing with what's going on, whereas I would just get the 'news updates'. I would often only get told the significant bits, and I would have to try and fill in the gaps for myself. But things were changing all the time. I used to feel like I was always playing catch up.

And I was never sure of my role. I felt like the others had their different roles, and sometimes I used to feel I was in the way a bit. When I came to visit and Dad was at home, there was little I could do, because my sisters and brothers had a routine, so I used to feel a bit like a spare part.

In the last three or four years of my father's life, I started to find a role. He started going into respite, for a week or two at a time, to give everyone else a break, and my role in those last few years was to go home at that time, and stay with my mum and spend time with her and look after her. She needed a level of care, so when I came over there was an opportunity for my brothers and sisters to take a complete break. And in a way that's a role I still continue with, since Dad died; I come over, and I step in, so that the others can step back if they want to.

I can see now that for all of us, my father's dementia had a different impact. Dementia affects everyone in the family in different ways. I was coming and going from the situation, whereas my mother and brothers and sisters were there all the time.

This whole thing about going backwards and forwards – I felt that the most when my father died. I got a text from my sister saying, 'Daddy's in hospital.' The doctors told my sister to tell the family that he may not last the night, so I went straight to Cork. My father lived for another week, in the hospital, and we took it in turns to be with him.

That week, and the days following his funeral, were probably the most challenging I've ever experienced. Going to the hospital and seeing my father, and knowing that he wasn't going to come out of this, and then going home to my mother, and having to tell my mother that my father wasn't coming home... That was a hard time.

We took my mum in to see him the day before he died, and it was heart-breaking. I looked and I saw the two people who fell in love and got married, spent all their years together, and now she was saying goodbye to him.

And when he did die, I felt like I didn't belong anywhere. I was staying in the house where I grew up, but it wasn't my own home any more, with my familiar things around me. I was aware that my brothers and sisters were able to take breaks from the intensity, because they were going home to their own homes and their own families – whereas I was staying in the house with my mother. Helen was there too. I'd have been lost without her.

And then when I came back to London, I was back in my own space – but here I was in a city that had no context for my father. Nobody knew him. He didn't know anything about my life here. So the loss was all the greater. I get sad because I feel he never really got to know Helen. He only began to get a sense of her, and of me living here in London, just as he started to become ill.

And afterwards, the first few visits home were just awful! I found it so hard! I came into the house – and Daddy wasn't there any more. I just couldn't settle. I can remember almost feeling, 'I can't bear being here.'

When he was in hospital in the last week of his life, he was on oxygen and a drip. He had become completely dehydrated, because he had stopped swallowing. When I visited him, I'd be holding his hand and stroking his forehead, and talking to him, saying, 'We're all right. We'll all be okay. You need to look after yourself now, and if you need to go, you go.' I knew that *for him*, the best thing was for him to die.

But *for me*, he could have stayed for as long as he wanted! People say, oh well, you were losing him for years, he didn't know who you were – it doesn't matter, he's your father, you still want him to be there. What people don't tell you, until it happens, is that when you lose a parent, it leaves a big hole that nothing else fills.

When you lose somebody to dementia, bit by bit, you can still put your hand out and touch them. They're still there. You can see them. It's a loss, but they're alive! When they actually die, it's final, and it's a big shock to the system. Some months after his death, the two losses – the loss of my father, when he died, and the loss of him for years and years to dementia – suddenly came together. And that was a fierce loss.

15

A Very Important Moustache

Steve Jeffery

My mother died on 5 January 2006, aged 96 and three-quarters. She had led a full and active life, physically and intellectually, for 90 of those years, including being a member of the executive of the Communist party, CND campaigner, mother, grandmother and great-grandmother. Then she started to get a little confused, then a little more, until, after about three falls at home that could not be explained, she was diagnosed with multi-infarct dementia. This is a progressive disorder with increasing loss of mental and bodily functions due to successions of 'small strokes' (tiny haemorrhages in the brain). At first the effects are not obvious: perhaps some confusion or getting a bit disorientated on what should be familiar routes. And to begin with I resisted my sister's diagnosis that these were the early signs of a dementing illness, taking refuge in the idea it was 'wear and tear'. But my sister's view from a distance was clearer, and when my mother had to be brought home from the high street by some kind strangers I had to admit I was wrong. Then came the falls, a spell in Lewisham Hospital, and finally the diagnosis. After a few months in hospital we found a nursing home for Mum nearby.

Multi-infarct dementia is a disorder which has little to recommend it, as you watch the person you love lose his or her memory, the ability to walk, and gradually the ability to talk and probably to understand. For the last two years of her life Mum had no speech at all. The only good thing in her case, and I have no idea if this is common in this form of dementia, is that she was rarely upset, and in the end died peacefully after two weeks of semi-consciousness.

Dementia robs both the sufferer and his or her carers of memory. For the person with dementia this begins with current memory, then past memory and finally all memory; for the carers it is the memory of who that person was which is gradually eroded. I can remember discussing with my brother or my wife and daughter how Nora was, and us saying, 'Not too bad today,'

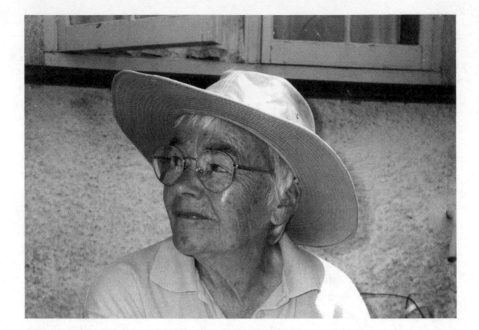

Nora Jeffery

which meant she might have said one word in an hour of mumbles, this being one word more than the week before. The norms of behaviour shift, and the pictures of the present for some reason blot out the past. Even though you try to take active steps to prevent this, it still happens.

I managed to rescue just a few tiny pieces from the wreckage, due to my obsessive habit of writing things down. I can get few positives from those last two years, but while Mum could speak, I realised that on many occasions she was being unintentionally funny, and at other times her unusual responses achieved more than normal speech. It helped that even though she knew things were not right, this knowledge did not distress her, and sometimes we would both end up with tears rolling down our cheeks. And, of course, I was always laughing with her, never at her.

I remember once asking what had happened to her that day, to be told: 'A man came in with a very important moustache.' On another occasion I was trying, without success, to explain something to her. When she finally gave up the attempt she announced: 'I must be losing my bonkers!' When I was trying to give her some exercise I asked her if she could walk. 'I don't think any of me could walk,' came the eloquent response.

Mum remembered her own mother long after she had forgotten who I was, and one day she told me, 'I'm worried about my mother.' I wasn't sure what to do, as she had been dead for nearly 50 years. I decided to be tactful.

'Mum, she's dead.'

'So what does that mean?'

I was completely stumped.

'Well, I'm 50, and when I was six your mum died. That's how long she's been dead.'

She fixed me with a long, hard look.

'I find that very hard to believe.'

'Well, it's true.'

'So tell me, as one individual to another, what do you think we can do for her?'

Mum had difficulty from the first in remembering names, especially mine and my grandson's, Reuben, so much so that Reuben became Rhubarb, until this was also forgotten. We were discussing Reuben one day when I asked Mum who his mother was. She shook her head. 'Should I know?'

I nodded.

'Don't know.'

I pointed at myself, as a clue to Rebecca, who is my daughter and Reuben's mother. Mum looked triumphant.

'You!'

'No, Mum, it has to be a woman.'

Still no joy, so I said, 'Rebecca.' Nothing. 'My daughter.' Still nothing.

I then wondered if she knew who I was.

'I know you, but you've a very unusual name, haven't you?'

'Well, you gave it to me.'

'No, I don't know.'

I was getting a little irritated by this point, which says more about me than my mother.

'How many children have you got?' I asked a bit curtly.

'Three.'

'And who are they?'

'David... Jill... and you.'

'And I am?'

'Asbestos!'

Gales of laughter. 'No, I wouldn't have called you that, would I?'

But I remained Asbestos for many weeks.

When discussing who was who in the family, Mum was surprised to find that I was married.

'It was one of *those* marriages was it?'

'What do you mean?'

'Married at nine or ten years old.'

I explained that I was married at eighteen.

'Well you must have been potty then.'

'Why?'

'Most people go potty through being married.'

A couple of days later my married status was still a cause for concern.

'Does anyone else know about this? If I tell Jill she'll be amazed.'

'I've been married for 32 years.'

'Does anyone else know?'

After a long explanation of how she had been at the wedding, Mum said: 'Is it a proper marriage with Iriss?'

'What do you mean?'

'With sex relationship?'

'Yes.'

Pause. 'I can hardly believe it.'

Sometimes, without meaning to be, I knew that I was being quite patronising, and so did she. She was wondering whether she could have a fold-up table in case someone came to tea, an event that sadly would never happen, when I said to her, 'Let's not cross that bridge till we come to it.' As it came out, I just knew it sounded pompous, but Mum's response gave me my comeuppance.

'And don't you be so snooty if you haven't got such a snoot!'

Even as I type this I can see my mother on these various occasions. She could still laugh at herself, and produce 'Alice through the Looking Glass' put-downs that could not possibly come to anyone with normal thought processes, that would bring tears to both our eyes.

The change in Mum's memories, and slow loss of recognition of those who loved her, meant that she altered as a person throughout the illness. So I suppose that she really ended as someone else, and in the end someone about whose thought processes I was completely in the dark. Despite this change and decline, for some of the time there was enough of her old self remaining, and enough of the changed person she was becoming, to give memories that are more happy than sad. I would advise anyone else who is a carer of someone in this condition to note down what you can while speech lasts, because it can tide you over while you wait for the glass of the past to clear and for memories of how people were to come flooding back. At least, that is my hope.

I would also caution to be careful of what you throw away. Photos are obviously important, but so far even those have not awoken my memories. But one of the things that had the strongest effect on me, I would have thrown away: my mother's long unused purse, stuck for six years in the bottom drawer of her bedside cabinet in the nursing home.

If my daughter hadn't rescued it from the bin, we would never have found the small piece of card tucked inside. On the front of the card was my mother's name, address and phone number; on the back the names of myself, my wife and my son and daughter. (We lived in the flat above her.) It was written by my daughter, when her grandmother told her she could no longer always remember who she was, or how she might get home. And that little piece of card reminded me of how we all loved each other and tried the best we could to deal with something so unbearable.[1]

Note

[1]   This article first appeared in the *Guardian*, 1 April 2006.

DESPATCHES FROM
THE BATTLEFIELD

16

This Has Gone Beyond my Mother

Marylyn Duncan

As told to Lucy Whitman.

I've been looking after my mum full-time for about five years. My mum is a very strong, determined woman. Sometimes I say she's bloody-minded, but probably being bloody-minded is what has seen her through to 88!

My mum was born in Tobago, but she moved to Trinidad, where I grew up. She has always been a very caring, hard-working person. She was a house-wife who took part in different projects in the community, including the women's group and village council. At home she planted vegetables, fruit trees, flowers and medicinal herbs and kept chickens. And she had a beautiful voice. She used to 'belt out' as my father described it, from the house. You could hear her for miles around. She just sang and sang. It was all hymns.

After my father died, in 1985, she used to come and spend six months with us, sometimes a year, and she enjoyed that because then she went back to her own community. In Trinidad, people would pass by and they would call out to her. There's always someone to speak to. While here, what she says is that you could be at home all day and not see anyone, so she didn't really like it here.

I think my mum's journey into dementia began when she started accus-ing people of taking her things. At first I believed her, but then I thought, 'But they wouldn't take her medication! They wouldn't take her clothing.' So alarm bells started going off. Then she came here, and started accusing us of taking her money, and accusing my son Anton's friends of taking her knick-ers. And I thought, 'Well no, my mum is a size 22. They can't be taking her knickers!'

Things gradually got worse, so I took her to the GP, who referred her to the memory clinic. The consultant explained what was going on and started her on Aricept. She did extremely well, and I thought it would be safe for her to go back to Trinidad. But when she was there, she hid her medication, apparently, and stopped taking it, so she deteriorated. I had to ask a neighbour to put her on a plane and send her back to London, and that was it.

Anton was just on the point of moving out when my mum came to live with us. But I said to him, 'Look, I can't carry this alone. Will you please not move out. I'm asking you to stay.' So he did. I have been lucky.

I still think that I didn't take it all on board, but then she started to hide everything in our house. You couldn't find anything. I had this habit of leaving my bills on the dining room table, to remind me to pay them in good time.

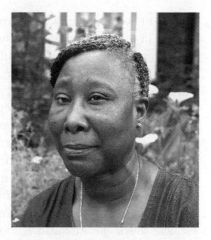

Marylyn Duncan © Helen Valentine helen@nakedeyeimages.co.uk

But what we didn't realise was, she was putting them back in the envelopes and filing them away in a drawer. So I had to pay interest for late bills.

She insisted on cooking, until one day Anton said to me, 'Please don't let Gran cook!' My mother was a beautiful cook. She'd come over here with all sorts of ingredients in her suitcases to try out recipes. When the dementia kicked in, she still insisted on cooking, but some of it was inedible, because she just could not remember how to cook. Before she got to that stage, she would say, 'I don't seem to be able to remember anything, write it down.' So I'd write notes before I left for work, and she would follow it. But then it came to the point, when you wrote it, she just folded it neatly and put it away.

My mum was an avid reader. She's not saying it so much now, but my mum was aware that she had lost her memory. She used to say to the doctors, 'When someone lose their memory, it is an *awful* thing.' But she can't retain anything. She doesn't read now.

Anton and I both came home, on different occasions, and found the house full of gas. I thought I was going to pass out. She was sitting there, watching TV, quarrelling with Anne Robinson, because she says she's so rude. And the house was full of gas. And I said to her, 'Mum, what are you doing? The house is stinking of gas.'

'Well, I can't smell any gas.'

That's when I decided, I couldn't work full-time any more. I am a mental health nurse, and I worked in the crisis team. First of all I went part-time.

They bent over backwards to help me at work. But I couldn't do it. I was getting up in the morning, I was rushing her, to get her medication, get her to the bathroom, do her breakfast. And then one morning, I just thought: Why am I doing this? I'm stressing her out, and I'm stressing myself out even more. I decided no. I couldn't swing it. I gave up work four years ago.

One day I took her to the doctor's for a check-up, and the GP took one look at me, and gave me this slip of paper with the number for the Admiral Nurse Service, and said I should contact them. So I was allocated an Admiral nurse, and she in turn contacted social services, and gave me the details of the local Alzheimer's Society support group. I had never claimed any benefits for my mum. Because I was working I just got on with it. I couldn't be bothered with the hassle of applying for anything. But they did the whole thing for me, and so she got Attendance Allowance.

The Admiral nurse was brilliant. I was very sceptical at first, but I warmed to her. I found that I can just bare my inmost soul to her, and not feel guilty. I can just tell her what's going on, how I feel. And I got that from the local Alzheimer's support group as well. You could go there, be with others in the same boat as you are, just talk and talk about what's happening with you, listen to other people's experiences and exchange suggestions and support.

My mother was pretty healthy, physically, until a few months ago, when she collapsed in the kitchen with a heart attack. We were bringing her back

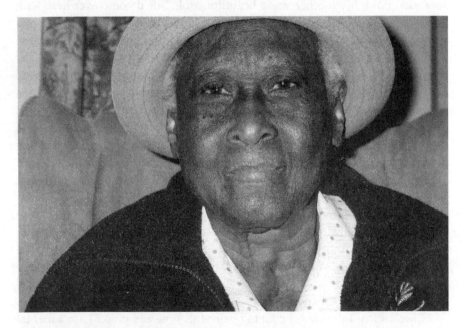

Marylyn's mother Camilla, better known as Queen

from the bathroom, and she literally dropped, like a fruit dropping from a tree. Her eyes rolled, her mouth went funny, and she was unconscious, and I actually thought she had died. Anton started to cry.

She was rushed to hospital 'on blue lights'. They thought we were losing her. I sat in the relatives' room with my son, and then his friends started coming in to find us. We talk about the young – and these are all male – but the network was fast. One of my friends also walked through the door, and stayed with me. That's when you know who your friends are.

I had this inner peace that my mum would survive. The consultants said to me, 'Your mother is critically ill. Did she ever express her wishes as to what she wanted to happen to her?'

I said to them, 'My mum's 88, she's not your frail elderly. She will pull through, she is strong. My mum comes from a family that live well into their nineties. Whatever needs doing, I expect you to do it for her, regardless of her age.'

And she did surprise them all. She pulled through.

The cardiologists eventually said they were convinced her heart attack was caused by the atenolol which she was taking for hypertension. I had informed her GP of an article I read in the *Daily Mail* that said atenolol could cause coronaries, but her response was, 'Oh, she's been on it a long time and it's keeping her blood pressure stable.' So she didn't want to change it.

Anyway, she pulled through, and she was transferred to the care of the elderly ward, for more tests, and that's where it all went pear-shaped.

When she arrived there, she became quite disorientated, and started picking at her clothing, something that she'd never done. Her whole behaviour changed, and I said to the staff nurse that I was concerned at my mother's mental state. And I got this real patronising answer: 'She's got dementia, so what do you expect?'

I said, 'Excuse me. Before my mum had a heart attack, she self-cared, with supervision. She could get about with the aid of a Zimmer frame, she was able to put in her own eye-drops, take herself to the bathroom, make herself a hot drink and a sandwich. What you're seeing here is not what my mother is like.'

It's the way she said it, as though, because she's got dementia, she's not a person! It made me think – this is a care of the elderly ward, and if that's the sort of response you get...

Then I saw something I had read about in the paper but had never thought I would see. Meals would be brought to the patients, put on the bedside locker, and then that would be it. I walked in one day. My mum was lying in bed, with cot-sides around her, lying flat, and her meal was on the bedside table beside her. From then on I decided to be there at mealtimes. I got her sitting at the edge of the bed, and after that, when the nurses saw what I was doing, they put her in a chair beside the bed, so she was able to feed herself.

There was this lady in the bed next to my mum. She was terribly confused, and literally just babbled. I said to her, 'Have your supper,' and another patient said to me, 'She can't feed herself. The nurses have to do it, and that depends on whether they have the time or not.' So I went over, and just talked her through it. 'Have a mouthful... well done... have another mouthful,' until she had eaten it all.

And then the medication – they put it in a little pot, put it next to them on their bedside table, and walk away. Yet this is a care of the elderly ward! What is going wrong in the NHS?

I went in there one time, and my mum was crying. She wanted to go to the toilet, and she said she was calling, waiting on someone to take her to the toilet. The added frustration was that she could see the toilet, but she couldn't get herself there. And her words were, 'When you have to rely on someone else to do things for you, it's a terrible thing.'

One day when I visited, my mum said to me that her heels felt as though they'd got sores on them. I mentioned it to the staff nurse who put a cushion-type dressing on both heels. That was on for about two days and then removed. She was also given an air mattress, initially, and that was removed. When I queried it, I was told that the tissue-viability nurse had assessed her, and decided that she didn't need it.

My mum was in a lot of pain. Her heels continued to shred, as you would shred paper, to the point where my mum, in her wisdom, said that mice were gnawing at her heels.

I pointed it out to the nurses, to the ward manager and the doctors, and asked what they were doing about it. I got no response, so I went down to the PALS office,[1] and they tried to set up a meeting between me, the ward manager and the tissue-viability nurse, to find out why the air mattress was removed. But that meeting never took place.

In the meantime, I went to a wedding in Tobago for two weeks. This had been arranged for over a year, and my son had agreed. Before I went, I asked where my mum would be when I got back. They told me she was too ill to be anywhere else but hospital. Yet while I was away, a nurse approached my son asking him to consider taking her home. He refused. He said his grandmother came under their care with unbroken skin, and that's how we expect to take her home.

I returned to smelly, oozy wounds on my mum's heels, one of which was without a dressing. It was just wrapped in ribbon-gauze and oozing on to the floor. And she didn't have an air mattress. So I went again, and spoke to the ward manager, and all she could tell me about was research. I was asking for some dressing or something to be put on it, but she was trying to tell me that that was an old-fashioned way of treating it. Years ago, you had to put a dressing on everything, but she said, 'Research shows that that's not necessary, you just leave it.'

I said to the ward manager, 'Every time I spoke to you, all you've told me about was research. But what system have you got in place, seeing as you've got all this research, to prevent what happened to my mother happening? You've never once told me.' So she was quiet.

I also said to her, 'I am doing this for all the others who are too scared to take issues on board and to challenge you, and also for those who have no one to fight their corner. This has gone beyond my mother. I've sat on this ward and watched what's going on.'

I went back to PALS, and saw the person I'd seen previously. She was incensed that the meeting with the tissue-viability nurse hadn't happened, and said she would lead an investigation to find out why. I said to her, 'We are past that now. I'm going to do a formal complaint.'

The consultant was in the room when I went and handed in the complaint. He was immediately given his copy, and read it, and came up to me and told me it was a nursing matter, not a clinical matter. However, shortly after, the air mattress went back on the bed.

The consultant asked for a meeting with me to discuss where my mum would go when she was discharged from hospital. And I said, 'Well, she's coming home. I've looked after her for all this time.' But I said this with the understanding that she would come home when her heels were healed. I didn't realise they were getting ready to put her out the door.

He then said to me I should think about it, because the physiotherapist has said that my mum wouldn't walk again. He said they have tried to walk her, and she hasn't been responding. And this is one of the stages of dementia, where they stop walking.

So I said to him, 'My mum has two holes where she should have heels. Don't you think that that makes a difference?'

Prior to that, my mum was going to be transferred to a rehabilitation unit, to get her mobilised again. But then the physiotherapist decided that she would never walk again, so the referral was not done. They said it wouldn't be appropriate to send her there.

He said to me that he was going to have a look at the heels, and I should phone him back to talk to him the next day. Then I spoke to my mum's GP. When I told her what was going on, she said she was very concerned because my mum must be in a lot of pain, and she wanted to know how they were managing the pain. She was also concerned because I told her the wound was smelly and she said that meant there were bacteria. She told me she would phone the consultant, and then the next day, instead of me phoning him, he phoned me. He said he had seen the wound, and prescribed a dressing; he was going to review it on a weekly basis, and he would contact me himself if there were any changes.

I told him I was determined that Mum was not coming home until her heels were healed, so don't even think about a discharge plan.

Then I received a phone call from a hoist company, saying they were due to install a hoist for my mother, who was being discharged on Monday! I said, 'Forget about the hoist. Just cancel it. I've done a formal complaint, and my mother is not coming home until her heels are healed.'

I then got on the phone to social services, and spoke to the discharge coordinator, who informed me that my mother had been in hospital for 89 days. My response was, 'My mother went into hospital with intact skin, and that's how she's going to come out. It's because of their neglect she's like this. And why can't she go to the rehabilitation unit?'

'The physiotherapist has said that she can't be rehabilitated.'

And I said, 'Four consultants told me that she wouldn't survive the heart attack, but she surprised them all. How can she walk, if she's got holes for heels?'

In the end, despite my daily visits, they discharged her on a Monday morning to a nursing home without informing me and gave my son the wrong number when we found out.

What a journey this has been. They tried their best to wear me down, especially at a case conference when there were six people against me. Fortunately, I had someone from the carers' group to accompany me.

The hospital eventually gave me an apology and invited me to become a patient advocate. I do believe I would take up the offer.

Note

[1]   The NHS Patient Advisory and Liaison Service, which has offices in many large hospitals and in some community centres. According to the PALS website, it exists 'to ensure that the NHS listens to patients, their relatives, carers and friends, and answers their questions and resolves their concerns as quickly as possible'. (www.pals.nhs.uk, accessed 24 March 2009).

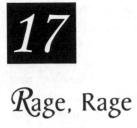

17

*R*age, Rage

Jenny Thomas

Dylan Thomas's famous poem 'Do not go gentle into that good night' exhorts us to rage against our diminishing life force.

When Mum's doctor told her that her expressionless face, muscle weakness and faltering feet meant that she had Parkinson's disease, did *she* rage?

Not at all. She accepted being unable to drive, social services adapting her home, meals on wheels and a weekly visit to a day centre with quiet dignity. The only thing she ever said which questioned her treatment was after her twentieth mini mental state test, you know the one, which asks: 'Who's the prime minister? Where do you live? What's the date? Remember these three words.'

'Do they think I'm stupid?' asked my 'mustn't grumble', acquiescent mum.

Then she fell in her kitchen and for the next six months she was too drugged and ill to rage. In any case, she would never have done so – she had never been ill before and she respectfully and gratefully put her complete trust in the NHS.

Did I rage for her? Well, yes. I researched, asked questions and tried everything I could from 180 miles away to restore her brain and body to normality.

I raged, but to little effect. Mum put her life in the hands of the NHS: the 'caring' profession, at all levels, rewarded her with uncaring, collective incompetence.

She entered hospital fully mobile and mentally bright, and left three and a half months later a doubly incontinent zombie in a wheelchair.

'Don't ever put me in a nursing home,' she had always said to me. But she needed 24-hour nursing care and two people and a hoist to move her.

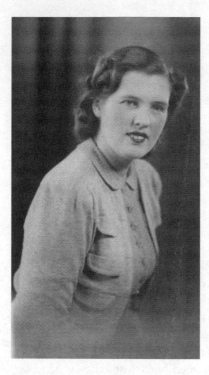

Jenny's mother Marjorie, c.1942

Research has shown that mice with dementia, kept in an enriched environment where they are stimulated mentally and physically, can learn new tasks, remember old ones and develop new brain cells. Yet every nursing home I saw stacked their inmates around a room with a TV blaring in the middle. No one was encouraged to talk, exercise or even walk. 'Hop in, Elsie, you're blocking the corridor.'

Life in a nursing home slowly, inexorably, dehumanises its residents. Having lost her home, her ability to walk, any control of her life and her confidence in her sharp brain, she then lost what she valued most – her dignity. What is it like to have no dignity? No self-esteem?

Even though it was written in her notes that she was to be washed and toileted by women only, my mum – who wouldn't enter a lavatory in her own house if there was anyone there to observe her doing so – was handled by men daily. I remember one particular example. Some relatives were visiting from America and Mum had been dressed in a beautiful, expensive frock which, before she went into hospital, she had been keeping for a special occasion. She was so nervous that she asked to go to the toilet, but instead of wheeling her into the one opposite, the two male carers pushed a commode into her room just as her visitors arrived. We waited outside until they brought out the uncovered receptacle and told us to go in. I rushed to open the window as we tried not to retch. Mum was deeply humiliated, mortified, the visit ruined.

At some point in the six months after she left hospital, it was decided that she had Lewy body dementia. This has the same symptoms as Parkinson's in its early stages. Lewy body dementia, unlike Alzheimer's, has fluctuating, intermittent symptoms; Mum's attention could change by the minute.

She was a clever, mentally active woman, who read newspapers daily and was interested in everyone and everything. But she was left to lie in bed for 18 out of every 24 hours, with nothing to do but dream. On some mornings she was still waiting to be got up for breakfast at 11 a.m. After two years, her bedsores became chronic, so it became 24 out of 24.

She could no longer read, as the words climbed on top of one another, and she was unable to change the channel on her blaring TV.

'Could you put the sound down?' Mum, with her perfect hearing, would beg every time I visited.

'Abandon hope, all ye who enter here,' is an apposite maxim for our experience of nursing care homes. She believed for two years that she was going to recover, ate everything she was offered and rested patiently, but I watched the hope dwindling away like the sand in an egg-timer.

Her teeth seemed to spend more time being re-lined and not being returned, than in her mouth. She looked and felt so much better when her hair was washed and set, and she had more than one bath a week – yet this was a weekly long-distance battle. Every time I visited, I found the £200 pressure cushion I had bought for her chair switched on, but on the floor and not under her – despite my notice on the wall and frequent talks with the staff.

I had to remember to check her medication every week. 'Why is she being given two different types of anti-depressants and two blood-thinning drugs?' Shouldn't relatives be informed when extra drugs are prescribed?

I checked her clothes every time, but all the better things disappeared and were never seen again. She had had 54 pairs of pants and 32 nighties and negligées with her when she moved in. I gave up with the pants when there were none left, as she no longer wore them on top of her capacious nappy. But why should she only have two faded old nighties? And where were all her lovely summer and winter suits, her dresses, rings, beautiful blouses, her cardigans – especially the two I knitted?

'Oh, don't worry, they'll come back,' Matron said comfortingly.

I learned not to leave chocolates and fruit, but feed them to her when there. Fruit rotted on her table and chocolates were eaten by the staff. Carers spooned her meals into her, but no extra.

Perhaps the tea saga was the single thing that made me most furious, because it could so easily have been changed. I asked and asked for a list of the residents' tea requirements to be put on the trolley. But no, it came five times a day, cold, too milky and with two sugars for everyone.

'Mum doesn't have milk, and only half a sugar,' I'd say every time, smiling politely.

Poor Mum. She slipped further and further away from me, from reality.

'This place is closing down next week,' she'd tell me.

'I could do with some runner beans. I've got a nice leg of pork to cook lunch for Beryl.'

Why did no one ever tell me that I shouldn't have corrected her when she said irrational things? Even a leaflet would have helped. I know now that I should have behaved as if she were being sensible.

'Am I talking rubbish *again?*' she'd ask.

I know it made her not want to speak.

She became a dried-up mummy, her hair and face devoid of colour, her hands cold claws which wouldn't straighten, her legs bruised sticks which wouldn't bend. She had shorter and fewer periods of lucidity. The reports from the staff grew less encouraging:

'Her bottom is too sore for her to sit out of bed.'

'She didn't want her hair washed this week.'

'Look at this scratch on my arm. She did that.'

Is Mum raging against this life at last? Is she trying to fight off the attentions of the carers? How could I know who did what? I lived and worked too far away and could only visit one or two days a week.

'What are these bruises all over her body?' I got no answers.

In the last two years of her life, her thinking and speaking rarely made a connection. She began a thought with the cues, the openers to conversations, but by the time she'd got through a few words, she'd forgotten where she was heading.

'I really think…'

'I think you should know…'

'Tell me, what do I do about this furl?'

'What's a furl, Mum?'

A wave of irritation at my stupidity passed across her skeletal face. Her ideas were flying about in threads and fragments. She knew at that moment that we weren't communicating and there was a desperate longing in her eyes to be understood.

Occasionally she showed flickers of animation. Glimmers of my mum lit up her features. Mostly she was dead-eyed, her lips shaping the same words, 'Help, help!' repeated over and over.

After four years, we rarely communicated. Being cut off from reality for so long, she was no longer interested in my world and could not explain hers to me. Did she know me?

'Of course,' she said.

But often my daughter and I had metamorphosed into one person. If she didn't know who people were, did she know who *she* was? Had she a sense of self? Without purpose in life and contact with reality, did the person she had always been become a distant memory? Was the mother I knew someone else?

Her life for six and a half years was my battleground. I fought for the best treatment for her, and mostly failed. Fought against the conditions in which she lived, and fought to keep her with me, as she slowly disappeared, bit by bit – so far away that I could no longer reach her. Her eyes were empty wells, her breath as fragile as glass threads, her nose a pointed beak and her skin like parchment stretched tight over her bones, which looked so sharp that they could have cut through the blanket covering them.

My experiences with Mum made me angry. Angry with myself for being unable to make the last years of her life better for her. Angry at the NHS for poor and uncaring treatment. Angry at the government for callous and inadequate funding and the lack of an integrated policy for health and social care. Angry at local authorities for their constant cut-backs, with social services for not providing clear information about entitlements.

And I am conscious that raging when one is old is too late, as age and illness bring fear, lack of confidence and resignation. We know that providing a life that every old person deserves would need a massive increase in funding, which would have to come from some other budget. Which one? Schools? Hospitals? No – no politicians would agree to this, as the very elderly rarely vote. So what will change the current system? If nothing else, surely it must be the selfishness of the baby boomer generation. If we want the best care for ourselves, we must start demanding it now.

Mum went gently. Can we?

Forever in my Thoughts

Rosie Smith

My father Ed died in 2006 at the age of 87. He had multi-infarct dementia, brought about by the mini-strokes he had suffered over the previous ten years.

He had always been a very jolly and affectionate man, and was a typical East End boy, having originated within the sound of Bow Bells. He was well-travelled from his days in the army in the Second World War, was very artistic, and had worked as a customs officer at Heathrow. My mum was three years his junior, and had been his loving wife since 1951.

At first my mum thought her husband's forgetfulness was due to old age, and assumed it was 'just what happens to us all', but he gradually became more and more dependent on her. Over several years, my mum soldiered on looking after Dad at home, and we all played our part in assisting them and taking them out. But Mum became exhausted with the 24/7 care demands. In the end, it reached a point when both physically and mentally, Mum could cope no more, and she collapsed with a breakdown.

My sisters and I all have our own young families and could not just stop everything to take care of him, so initially Dad went into respite care. However, Mum was assessed as clinically depressed; she needed three weeks in hospital on sedatives and various drugs before surfacing to face the world again.

While Mum was in hospital, Dad was transferred by the local authority to a registered nursing home, where he stayed until just before his death. Had we known then what we know now, we would have moved him after those first few weeks. He survived for one and a half years, and his deterioration seemed far more rapid than when 'kept going' by Mum at home.

To be elderly and ill is bad enough, but to be mentally impaired and elderly is terrible for the way that you are treated. The indignity of being in a care home where Dad would so often appear in other people's clothes, and thus lose so much more of his identity through no fault of his own, was heartbreaking for all of us. Dementia alone does a good job of changing someone, without social services adding to it! An image forever in my thoughts is of Dad advancing down the corridor towards me, dressed in someone else's too short jogging pants, hair cut as if in a concentration camp and wearing someone else's shirt.

To add insult to injury, he was expected to pay for most of the cost of his care from his own savings. This makes me livid, especially as I felt that they did not look after him properly.

Part of my concern for my father was that he may have suffered physical abuse, in addition to neglect. He frequently had bruising to face, legs and arms. When an explanation was sought, it was never more than, 'He had a fall.' The fact that he flinched once, when I went to stroke his hair, worried me, as in all the time I had helped to care for him, not once had that ever happened; it placed grave thoughts in my head regarding rough handling or worse.

I knew about the tendency for people with dementia to fall – as indeed with elderly persons in general – but I couldn't get the thought out of my head that possibly Dad was trying to get away, or find us or go for help.

We were very concerned when the care home suggested strapping him into a wheelchair to stop him from falling and hurting himself. I spoke with the manager who said that there were alternatives, such as special chairs they cannot get out of. I remember saying to her at the time, surely that is still restraint, and I'd far rather his needs be checked first to ensure he didn't want to get up for any reason. Also, why shouldn't he have someone to walk him about now and then, as I did with him whenever I could. Many weeks later, the elder abuse team got in touch with us, and started to investigate my large file of letters, but by that time my dad had died.

He was taken into hospital, at my intervention, with severe dehydration, and died two weeks later. Although it said on the death certificate 'heart failure', I remain convinced he actually died due to malnourishment and lack of fluids. I am aware that people with dementia often experience feeding difficulties and eventually lose the desire to eat, but I knew that he still had an interest in food and drink. However, it took much patience and time, something I believe the home did not offer consistently. He could not tell you verbally in those later times, yet through his eyes, facial expressions and actions it was possible for him to make his needs known. The sad truth is that it took someone to really know his signs, in order to recognise and, hence, meet his needs. I strongly believe that he met a premature end, and that he could have continued in better health for somewhat longer if he had received adequate care. As you can imagine, this kind of thing never leaves you.

In his final days at the hospital, he kissed my mum when she leant over to try and hear him. Then he did the same to me. We were both overcome with emotion and the realisation that he really did know how much we cared for him and just how much we loved him. It was his last touching goodbye and proved to me without a doubt that care homes miss much of a person and do not do enough to try to keep in contact with the person within. Many care-providers are sorely lacking in true understanding of their charges, especially when it comes to communication with the patient. My sister once likened his condition to a cloth placed over a lamp; the light is still there but somewhat masked.

Ed is very sorely missed by my dear mum and all his three daughters and our families. Although I had read up and knew what end-stage dementia can be like, I was not prepared for the feeling of hurt that he could have had better care for that final year and a half. My mum did such a good job, well into her eighties, keeping him going for so long and caring for him with such love.[1]

Note

[1]   Names have been changed.

19

A Sister's Story

Peggy Fray

My sister, Kathleen Anne Richards, was born on 15 July 1927: the feast of St Swithin – and not a drop of rain in sight. It was a lovely summer's day, one week before my fourth birthday.

Although I did not know it then, Kathleen had arrived with Down's syndrome, at the time more generally termed 'mongolism'. Families with a child with the condition then had two choices: either the child remained at home without formal support – and there was then no NHS and no benefits system – or the child would be placed in a large institution, sometimes far from the family home.

When she was six months old, a doctor told our mother that Kathleen would never walk or talk, or perhaps even sit up. He said our mother would be well advised to leave Kathleen with them, try to forget about her, and be thankful that she had one healthy child. Our mother's response was that Kathleen was her daughter, and she would care for her.

In those days, the estimated life span for a child with this condition was just nine years, yet Kathleen lived into her seventieth year. So, all unknowing, our mother began what became a lifetime of loving caring for Kathleen.

In 1933, aged six, Kathleen was refused admission to school by the local authority, which judged that children with Down's syndrome were ineducable. Apart from the death of her own father, this was the only time I saw our mother cry. However, just as earlier she had helped Kathleen to speak, her only tool a looking glass, so now our indomitable mother began the education of Kathleen, again without formal support. In time, Kathleen learned to read and write, to knit and sew, to embroider and paint, and to acquire all those ordinary everyday skills the rest of us take for granted.

Throughout these earlier years, Kathleen endured many painful infections. Whatever today's view of antibiotics may be, their advent following the war

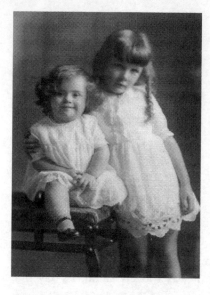

Peggy and Kathleen, 1931

years was an absolute boon for Kathleen and others with Down's syndrome.

Kathleen developed into a sensitive, warm-hearted, compassionate character, with a delightful sense of humour. Music was her greatest joy, and her lasting ambition was to sing and dance on the stage, inspired by the films of her early role model – Shirley Temple. Today, doubtless, she would have achieved that by joining one of the excellent groups of people with Down's syndrome who now entertain at events across the country. Sadly, there were none in Kathleen's era.

Kathleen did not like to be alone. Her favourite word was *together*. Everything should be done *together*. I shall always remember that when my young fiancé, an RAF Spitfire pilot, was killed in 1942, it was my little sister who put her arms around me in the night saying, 'Don't cry, Peggy, don't cry.'

This then was the young lady whom doctors had once predicted might never even sit up.

In 1959 our father died, and Kathleen and our mother came to live with me in a suburb of Preston. I nursed our mother at home when she became gravely ill, so that we could all stay together. When she died, in 1977, Kathleen and I comforted each other in our loss. Kathleen and our mother had never been apart for 50 years.

A few weeks later, we were out walking when Kathleen suddenly asked, very clearly, 'Peggy, what will happen to me, if anything happens to you?' I was utterly shocked. I had thought that this worry was mine alone – I had not given Kathleen credit for such foresight. It is clear to me that people with a learning disability know far more than most of us realise. I felt a huge surge of love for her, as I knew the depth of thought that had gone into producing that very concise question. I believe that I was able to reassure her, for the subject never arose again. It remained with me, however, where it had always been, in the back of my mind.

One evening in 1985, when Kathleen was 58, we had just returned home from a holiday when Kathleen suddenly collapsed. At hospital the doctor said that it was not a heart attack, but was probably the result of exhaustion from the long journey.

There is a recognised association between Down's syndrome and the risk of developing Alzheimer's disease,[1] but at this time I knew very little about it. Much later I realised that the collapse had probably been a mild stroke, because from then on Kathleen began to lean to her left side continually when seated. Her various activities began to deteriorate – for example, her knitting started to 'go wrong'. For quite some time I did not connect these failings with the collapse, and when I spoke to the doctor, she said it was just part of the ageing process. As time went on, however, it became apparent that Alzheimer's was taking hold.

In 1989 Kathleen developed a severe viral infection. She seemed to be recovering well, when suddenly, overnight, she became doubly incontinent, with total loss of all mobility, quickly followed by loss of speech. District nurses came in for twenty minutes twice a day, but Kathleen screamed whenever they moved her. At the end of six weeks, I knew I was defeated. The doctor said that if I did not let Kathleen go into hospital, she would soon be in one and I in another. I believe that Kathleen and I were both in a state of shock and devastation at this sudden loss of all her hard-won capabilities.

The doctor took me to visit a local community hospital where a bed was available and asked me to give her my decision the next morning.

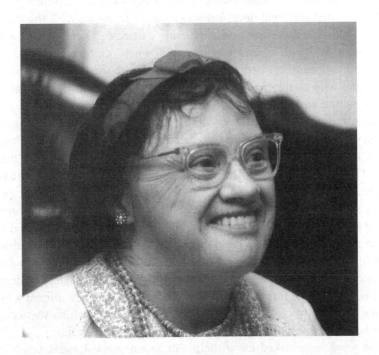

Kathleen, 1982

All night, in between attending to Kathleen, I roamed the house, trying to decide what was best. Since nursing our mother, I had found more comfort in poetry than in prayer, and now some lines of verse by Robert Frost kept running through my mind:

> The woods are lovely, dark and deep.
> But I have promises to keep,
> And miles to go before I sleep,
> And miles to go before I sleep.[2]

I was thinking of the promises I had made to our parents, to Kathleen, and to myself, that I would always take care of her. Now here I was, thinking of breaking those promises.

Finally, I decided that since there was only myself left to care for her, it would be better for her to be in safe hands in case I should die before her. At that time an NHS community hospital seemed to be the safest haven. It was a soul-destroying decision to have to make, for I loved her so deeply.

When the ambulance came, I went in beside Kathleen. After weeks of silence, she lifted her head, and in a firm, clear voice said, 'Goodbye.' So she did know what was happening. From then on, she virtually never spoke again. Neither of us ever cried again either; it was a sadness too deep for tears.

The hospital staff had never before cared for someone with the dual disability of Down's syndrome and Alzheimer's disease. There ensued a series of very stressful incidents and misdiagnoses, where Kathleen endured severe discomfort and unrecognised pain. This was despite the best efforts of good, kind nurses who simply had not been trained to deal with the special needs of those with Kathleen's condition.

Some months later, Kathleen developed severe epilepsy and also suffered several mini-strokes, which left her profoundly disabled. The hospital authorities began to put pressure upon me to remove Kathleen to a nursing home. This was at the time when long-stay beds in NHS hospitals were being systematically closed down, without making adequate provision for people such as Kathleen who had multiple disabilities and complex nursing needs. I applied to every home with nursing facilities for people with learning disabilities across the county. All declared they were 'crammed to the doors' through the influx of patients from the ongoing closure of the large mental handicap institutions in line with the new Community Care Act. Ultimately, in desperation, I sought advice from our MP. Two weeks later we were offered a bed in another community hospital, several miles further away, which we accepted. So we had to start all over again, with different hospital staff.

The ward sister asked me to help. For seven years, I spent seven hours every day with Kathleen, to help where I could, and just to be with her. Apart, that is, from three weeks, when I had treatment for cancer of the tongue. When told the tumour was malignant, my instinctive response was, 'Well, I can't die yet, I've got a little sister to look after.' At first I feared that I would lose my tongue, and be unable to speak to or for Kathleen, when she had already lost her speech.

Sadly, the dementia also reduced Kathleen's immune system, and she suffered constantly from recurring infections which caused her agonising pain, despite treatment, in her final years.

The physical nursing care that Kathleen received was faultless. Her person and her bed were always sweet and spotless. If any redness appeared on her skin she was moved every two hours, night and day, until it disappeared. Despite the extreme sensitivity of her skin, and being immobile for seven years, she never developed a pressure sore. Today, there is just a grassy plot where the hospital once stood, and those excellent nursing teams have disappeared with it.

Kathleen came to the end of her long journey on 6 February 1997.

Two months later, I discovered that there was a local community learning disability nursing team – who might have helped me look after Kathleen at home – yet Kathleen had been in hospital for seven years, and I had been there every day too.

After Kathleen's death, I found some private notebooks she had kept, in which she had written, at the top of every page, part of one of two words, leaving the rest of the page blank. The part words were HOSP and BOAR which I knew to be 'hospital' and 'Boarbank' – a large convent nursing home near our childhood village. Kathleen knew that these were places where people went to be made well again.

I had never talked to her about the various lapses she had had in her last years at home; I had just comforted her at the time, and hoped she would forget them. I had not realised how frightened she must have been as her capabilities deserted her. These pages were her cry for help – and no one had heard. She had not had the vocabulary to tell me that she knew something was wrong with her and she wanted to be made better. Looking at those pages, I was heartbroken.

That is why I now believe so strongly that everyone with a learning disability should have a personal health plan, and that people with Down's syndrome should have regular, sensitively administered assessments from at least the age of 30, not only that any changes may be noted, but just as importantly, so that the individual may speak about any concerns he or she may have. No one should be left alone with the loneliness that my sister must have experienced, despite my great love for her.

For a long time after Kathleen left, I was lost and angry – lost without her, angry at the way this cruel illness had stripped her of all the hard-won capabilities which she had struggled with such determination to achieve, angry at the silent suffering of those seven long years, and angry at the lack of knowledge and lack of training – both about learning disability and dementia – amongst many health professionals and support workers. Our mother would have counselled acceptance, but I never could find my way there. If God is good, I thought, how could the innocent suffer like this?

Lately however, as I sit quietly working in my room, I sometimes become aware of what I can only describe as a warm glow spreading around, and I know it is Kathleen's brave spirit letting me know she is there; with that has come a sort of peace.

For many young people with Down's syndrome today, the opportunities and lifestyle that lie before them are so vastly different from the bleak prospect that confronted Kathleen and those of her era. It is difficult to believe that such a great improvement could have taken place in one woman's lifetime, but thankfully it has. Despite that, there is still a long way to go. One only has to read the Mencap report *Death by Indifference*[3] – which shows how even today, people with learning disabilities are sometimes denied life-saving treatment – to know that the fight must continue.

I believe that all of us – people with a learning disability, their families and carers, statutory services, voluntary organisations and the Standing Commission on Carers – have a responsibility to work *together* (to quote Kathleen's favourite word) towards an even better future for people with a learning disability.[4]

Notes

[1]   See *Down's Syndrome and Alzheimer's Disease: A Guide for Parents and Carers* (2004) Teddington: Down's Syndrome Association. Available free from the Down's Syndrome Association on 0845 230 0372 or download at www.downs-syndrome.org.uk/resources/publications/medical-and-health.html, accessed 26 March 2009.

[2]   Frost, R. (1923) 'Stopping by woods on a snowy evening.' In R. Frost (1998) *Selected Poems*. Adrian Barlow (ed.). Oxford: OUP, p.41.

[3]   Mencap (2007) *Death by Indifference*. London: Mencap. Available from Mencap on 020 7454 0454, or download from www.mencap.org.uk, accessed via the Resources link, 26 March 2009.

[4]   Peggy Fray's story of looking after her sister is told at greater length in her book *Caring for Kathleen*. Fray, Margaret T. (2000) *Caring for Kathleen*. Kidderminster: BILD Publications.

20

Surely the World has Changed?

Roger Newman

To begin at the end of the story. My partner had a very virulent form of Alzheimer's disease, and had been living in a residential home very close to our house for nearly six years. The home met his needs in a remarkable way, bearing in mind the challenging nature of his behaviour. I continued with my job, but visited him each day to give him some tender loving care. I usually brought him down to our house, where we could spend quality time together. One lunchtime, he suddenly went missing from the residential home. After 24 hours of searching, he was found dead on the beach. He was 62, and had been diagnosed with the condition for eight years.

My experiences of caring for someone with dementia were similar to those of other carers: the feelings of helplessness, frustration at the inability to communicate easily, exhaustion, guilt, isolation, and the realisation of how it would eventually end, were all present in my mind on a daily basis. Above all, I had that feeling of devotion for a person who had been with me for 30 years, with whom I had made love, shopped, cooked, gardened, socialised, discussed and argued.

David and I had been through a lot in order to be together. We were both children of an age when being gay had been as difficult as it could be. Neither of us in our teenage years had really understood the feelings which were embedded in us, and both of us, for good and understandable reasons, had married. In order to be together, we had later left our wives, who experienced all the trauma and hurt created by those actions.

So we became a gay couple, 'out' to those we felt safe with, and an enigma to those whose positive reactions to our truth could not be counted on. We were able to create a good lifestyle and to surround ourselves with people and things which gave us a feeling of security and permanence.

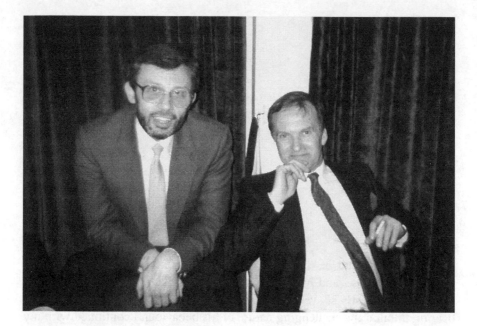

Roger (left) with David, 1987

When David's behaviour started to show signs of a fundamental change, it didn't take long before that well-established pattern of our lives began to fall apart. We had built a wall around our relationship which made us feel that it was easy being a gay couple and we truly believed that that was how it was going to be. The onset of David's dementia, however, turned every-thing upside down. For a start, having no expectation that dementia could hit someone of 52, and in any case, having no real knowledge of the condition, my first reaction to his changed behaviour was to feel that he had decided that the relationship was over, and consequently I left him. When later I real-ised that something more serious was happening to him, I knew that I wanted to assume a caring role: our twenty years together could not be discounted that easily. However, having to deal with people not in 'our circle' meant that those walls we had carefully built now had to allow for some breaches in them so that we could be helped. Sadly, at times, the professionals who walked through those gaps weren't always understanding of our situation nor did they make us feel as safe as we would have liked. Some doctors would not accept my role, or the validity of our relationship, without me having to be quite forceful in my reactions. As the dementia took hold, David aged visibly, and some people just assumed that he was my father. I did not want to let such a misunderstanding go, and I always felt it necessary to say that he was my partner. Life soon became an endless sequence of 'coming out' to anyone who dealt with us, but I didn't worry about this since it seemed best in order to ensure that David would receive the best care possible.

In the residential home, at the beginning, they didn't quite grasp the implications of me being his partner and not just a close friend. There were too many times when I was told about a social services or medical appointment at the last moment, making it difficult to change my work plans. I had to say quite pointedly that nothing should be arranged without first informing me. Eventually, this understanding was established and they soon learned its value, when flu injections, or visits from the chiropodist, or the need to trim his moustache could not be completed without my smiling face calming him, and without me holding him quite firmly to ensure a successful result.

David did not have the same inhibitions about our relationship or his sexuality as I had, as his carer. When we went out for a walk or went shopping I dreaded those moments when I knew he would want to go to the toilet because his smiles and knowing looks at other men spelled such potential danger that I feared he could be attacked before I had the chance to explain his condition. Similarly, he had no inhibitions about showing affection in public, and so he now kissed me frequently, wherever we might be. I was faced with a challenge – should I respond positively to the person I loved, or attempt a cover-up, to try to avoid the reactions of those who were not used to seeing two men kissing? I quickly decided who came first, and accepted whatever consequences might follow.

I began to realise that both of us were now in a world which was far and away different from the world we had created. In the good old days, we chose where we would go and who we would be associated with. If a situation was not to our liking, or if we found ourselves with people who seemed unsympathetic to our sexuality and lifestyle, it was easy to withdraw back into the safety of our home and the company of people we loved and trusted. Our house and friends and family were the walls which protected us from those outside who were less sympathetic to homosexuality. Once David was in residential care, we entered a world where everyone seemed either to be husband, wife or single, and much of our feeling of security vanished. Gone were those times when we could go to the gay disco; or phone our friends and camp it up with our conversation; or have visitors and greet them lovingly and physically; or have our gay magazines around us; or watch those TV programmes which were clearly for gay viewers. When David needed to be cuddled, I felt we had to go to his room to do it.

Yes, everyone was kind and friendly in the residential home. Yes, I frequently stayed and had food with him and was welcomed. Yet I was never able to get rid of the feeling that these were just not our people! Something inside me made me feel deeply psychologically unsafe because I suddenly realised how much he and I had relied upon other members of our gay community for our wellbeing and happiness. Yes, gay friends and lovely straight friends did visit us in that home, but as soon as they entered, a large amount of the openness which we had thrived upon was lost and they too seemed to feel insecure. The hugs lost their physical closeness, the humour lost its raunchiness, the conversation lost its knowingness because we were no longer in a 'family' environment.

I did my best to try to change things. When David was 60, I decided that we would have a celebration, not at our house, but instead in the care home, and our gay friends would be invited. They all turned up, the staff at the home decorated David's spacious accommodation, and things went well. I shall always remember David singing 'Happy Birthday' with the rest of us, presumably because he still remembered the words but couldn't remember why he was singing them, and while the rest of us ate our sandwiches and cake, he got into bed, seemingly rather glad that he had such a lot of people to sleep with that night! Nevertheless, all that well-meaning activity did not alleviate those feelings of being lost in another world.

When David and I set up home together, we tended to count the success of our relationship on the basis of what we owned and what things we did together. Almost immediately, in 1970, we had set up a joint bank account, to the bemusement of our bank manager who naively assumed that we were running a business in addition to doing our other jobs. We then negotiated a joint mortgage and at the time must have been one of the first gay couples to do so. The building society manager seemed to think that two men making such an arrangement carried more risk than a heterosexual couple, and needed reminding that the soaring divorce rate didn't quite validate his views. We were spending our increasing salaries as if there were no tomorrow; we had bought a second home and enjoyed frequent holidays. We never sat down to work out a contract about the boundaries of our behaviour and we had not made promises about being faithful. By the time the AIDS pandemic arrived in the 1980s, the pattern of our relationship was already firmly established and we knew that we just had to be more careful. With the onset of David's dementia that pattern was thrown into confusion. His sexual behaviour became more extreme, and as I have said, I felt damaged and left him.

When the full nature of his profound dementia became clear and when more service providers were involved, I realised that something was happening to people's attitudes to us both. We now merited the label of being an established and stable couple. I felt, however, that we were being given the role of an honorary straight couple, and that all the assumptions surrounding heterosexual activity were now being offloaded onto us. David was referred to as 'the love of my life' – and indeed, we had been together for a long time and we did love each other – but we were gay and needed to be treated with an understanding of what gay couples thought and did.

I never stopped loving David, but I desperately wanted the gap created by this terrible illness filled. Once or twice, during the early stages of his illness, I tried to have sex with him, but I knew that it was for my benefit that it was happening and I felt no comfort or satisfaction but only a load of guilt that I might have been using him. So, after three years, I looked for someone new to enter my life and to my surprise found a new lover, Michael, who lived not too far away. We made clear contracts about our behaviour and how caring for David would figure in our lives. There was never any doubt that David's needs would come first, and we made our decision gladly and without regret. Michael provided all the support I could possibly need, though I know that he felt some guilt when in David's presence. His support was invaluable, not least during those terrible days following David's disappearance and death. At David's funeral, we celebrated his life, his very real qualities and our life together, but I felt there was to be no fudging about the past and no embarrassment either about my present situation. Michael sat next to me throughout the service, as did David's family, and some of our many gay friends.

What does all this mean now, some eight years after David's death? Well, certainly the trauma arising from David's disappearance has had an effect which continues to this day. When I dream, whatever the subject, David's disappearance suddenly intrudes, and I experience the panic and pain of those hours once more. It might be a perfectly delightful dream, but it is interrupted by the loss of David. At first it happened every night, but it is less frequent now. I presume the memory of that time will never completely go.

Like all people who have been carers, I find that all sorts of things trigger the memory and that gut-wrenching, deep sadness takes over. Towards the end of his life, there were very few things which David could still say, but for some reason he still remembered the words of the song, 'You are my sunshine, my only sunshine'. Hardly a day went by that I didn't test him on those words and I always hugged him after he had got them correct again. I shall always remember the look of childlike pride on his face after he had said them.

Time spent with him always contained sustained mutual eye contact, and a smile on my face, as I said slowly, and he whispered with me, 'I love you.' Although, even now, I feel the pain of those times, there is also deep comfort in the knowledge that in his world of confusion and memory loss, he knew that in my presence there was security and protection.

No one emerges from dementia care without a huge fund of knowledge and experience about the condition, and as a former carer I have tried to use all of that for the benefit of those whose journeys are just starting. I am active in my local Alzheimer's Society branch, and I meet many men, both gay and straight, who are experiencing loss and confusion as they struggle to provide care for loved ones with dementia. Male carers have a lot to learn when their journey begins, and require an empathic closeness where they can offload their feelings without an accompanying sense of betraying their masculinity. In the right circumstances and in a measured way, they can benefit from the concern of a gay man who has learned to be close to other men without feeling threatened.

I am also a founder member of the Alzheimer's Society LGBT (lesbian, gay, bisexual and transgender) carers' group. When I first joined the Alzheimer's Society, soon after David was diagnosed in 1995, I felt very frustrated by the apparent assumption – in the society's monthly magazine and its other literature – that the disease only affected married couples or those with supportive families. The focus seemed to be on heroic husbands or wives, married for scores of years, or devoted sons and daughters. There were no examples of people in other kinds of relationships. It was difficult for me to identify with such images or to incorporate them into my experience as a carer. I wrote a letter to the magazine, explaining that these assumptions made it hard for me to feel welcome in the organisation, and pointing out that the society had failed to recognise the particular needs and experiences of lesbian and gay carers. Other members responded to my letter, and the network came into being.

Some people said to us from the outset, 'Surely the world has changed in its attitude towards you, and the law has followed suit? Why do you need something special when society is already more sympathetic?' They do not realise that older gay men and lesbians bring with us, to this task of caring, a significant amount of baggage from a previous age. The men remember all too clearly being 'illegal' and being victims of police harassment. The women remember a society where people hardly believed that lesbians actually existed. All of us have a past knowledge of beatings, murder and discrimination in the workplace, and over the years – as I have described above – we have learned to build protective walls around our lives, making us relatively anonymous and giving us the maximum feeling of safety. But a new and threatening world suddenly arises for the 60- or 70-year-old gay carer who has to divulge his or her personal circumstances at the hospital, the doctor's surgery, or on the phone to a social worker, and this all happens at a time when the pressure, emotion and isolation of being a carer can be at its greatest.

To its credit, the Alzheimer's Society has taken these issues on board in an impressive way. The LGBT group has its own pages on the society's website, receiving hundreds of hits per month, and providing vitally important recognition, acknowledgement and understanding, as well as useful information, for lesbian and gay carers.[1] Over the years, a variety of health and social service professionals have contacted us, usually with an admission that it had not previously occurred to them that lesbian and gay carers might have unique and unmet needs. We have been invited to speak at numerous meetings and conferences, and the resulting changes in practice and awareness have been extraordinary.[2] However, there remains a deep need within the health and social services sector to learn more about us as gay people, to learn how to empathise so that we feel safe to talk about our relationships and our needs, and to encourage us to request help without feeling threatened.[3] When society achieves that, the need for an LGBT network will decrease, but we all know that we are a long way from that goal at present.

A few days before David died, I brought him down to our house as usual and, also as usual, in the hall, having taken off his coat, we hugged and kissed. For some reason, on that day, I said to him, 'Oh, I don't want to lose you just yet.' That may have been almost the last thing I said to him. In many ways, I hope it was. Like all carers, I had long accepted the inevitability of what the end of this terrible illness would be, but my feelings about David had transcended the huge demands of caring, and I was willing to continue meeting those demands, however long it took. I am so grateful for having had to do that.[4]

Notes

[1] See www.alzheimers.org.uk/gaycarers (accessed 26 March 2009) or phone 0845 300 0336 for further information.

[2] See for example, Commission for Social Care Inspection (2008) *Putting People First: Equality and Diversity Matters 1: Providing Appropriate Services for Lesbian, Gay and Bisexual and Transgender People.* Available at www.cqc.org.uk/_db/_documents/putting_people_first_equality_and_diversity_matters_1.pdf, accessed 6 May 2009. Printed copies available free on request on 0870 240 7535.

[3] Useful resources are available from Age Concern England's Opening Doors project at www.ageconcern.org.uk/AgeConcern/openingdoors_about.asp, accessed 26 March 2009.

[4] Some of the material in this chapter first appeared in Newman, R. (2005) 'Partners in care – Being equally different: lesbian and gay carers.' *Psychiatric Bulletin 29*, 266–269.

21

Look Back in Anger

Shirley Nurock

Looking back, it seems hard to believe that my 'caring career' started over twenty years ago. In spite of the horrors of Alzheimer's as endured by my husband on his sixteen-year journey, and the distress and anguish experienced by our family, somewhat to my surprise, I am still here to tell his tale and, more importantly, pursue the battle for better services and recognition for people with dementia.

In 1994, I described my family's experience in two articles published in the Alzheimer's Disease Society newsletter. I wrote:

> My husband was a doctor – a GP in a large south London practice for over 30 years. He was diagnosed some five years ago as a younger sufferer from Alzheimer's disease.
>
> The diagnosis was such a shock to him that he never set foot in his surgery or drove a car again. He was given no follow-up by a consultant, nor offered any professional emotional support. Just the diagnosis and 'There's nothing we can do – try and keep as healthy as possible.' He knew and I knew that there was no cure, but can you imagine the impact the diagnosis had on him as a doctor himself? In a way he felt humiliated. Surely, Alzheimer's disease could be classed as extreme as cancer – and yet an Alzheimer's sufferer is almost universally shunned by the medical profession.
>
> Perhaps a doctor is simply expected to be braver than anyone else. In the early stages he was distressingly aware of the situation but tried to hide his feelings, just as he hid his feelings from patients when upset by their diseases. But he was still able to be an understanding and caring professional. How welcome a few words of sympathy from a GP or a consultant would have been then.

Being a 'young' sufferer presented its own problems. He was too young to be referred to a psychogeriatrician and not required to be visited by the GP. Nowhere could I make contact with other young sufferers at a similar stage of the disease to meet with him for company. Physically he was very fit and active, hopelessly out of place in the local day centre, and I wouldn't let him go there. No remotely suitable day care or respite care was or is available. Perhaps it was not surprising that he became very depressed early on in the disease.

As I struggled with my own emotional turmoil and faced the social and financial implications for the future, I had, and still have, the feeling that it need not have been like this. Certainly my own grieving process would not have been stuck permanently in this stage of anger if things had been different. Is it so hard for a consultant to follow up such a patient or to be seen to care? An expression of concern at his deteriorating state, or of encouragement, could have helped him. Not like the consultant who abruptly told me how bad my husband's memory was and refused to believe he could still have feelings...

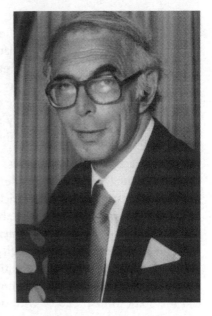

Leonard Nurock, 1988, early stage Alzheimer's

How does the wife in her forties ever come to terms with the loss of a loved partner? Gone the shared memories, shared happiness, the future you had planned together. What remains? Coping with the practical aspects of bringing up a family, working and caring for a husband, planning for a future which you don't want to happen, with its social, financial and legal burdens. To bear the hurt of friends and family who vanish into thin air, the humiliation of always being dependent on others, the isolation of caring, this nightmare that nothing could have ever really prepared you for. To find the strength to battle for advice on caring, support, the benefits and services available – those services which never catch up with your needs. Alzheimer's is not a static illness. It requires continuous reassessment.

How to come to terms with the emotional side of the long bereavement? Anger – or grief masked as anger – guilt, depression, despair, frustration, numbness, disbelief, agony and ultimately, horror as the disease progresses at a furious pace and you are forced into the role of bystander, overcome by the realisation of how ill you feel from stress and how deeply affected by pity and heart-rending sorrow at what is happening to this man...

How do children view the gradual loss of a father, he who they barely had time to know as he once was, for they have grown up with his increasing vagueness and forgetfulness? He cannot help with their homework or share in their successes – instead they must feed him. But his illness must not be allowed to stand in the way of their paths to independence...[1]

Over the years, increased awareness has prompted improvements in care, but sadly the stigma and ageist attitudes still predominate. In spite of an increase in funds for research, it is still a fraction of that spent on other major diseases and totally disproportionate to the huge burden of costs that dementia places upon society and individuals. Dementia is still not seen as a priority.

The development and availability, if you are lucky, of anti-dementia drugs is a step forward, as is the recognition through research of better care pathways, services and treatments. We now understand the potential of psychological therapies to help people with dementia and their carers, and how levels of care both in the community and in care homes can be optimised. Younger people with dementia are now a recognised group. Twenty years ago this was not the case and there were no appropriate services for my husband.

Researchers and carers know the answers, yet there are still tens of thousands of distraught carers out there, struggling along without support, as local councils are forced to cut back their social care budgets to the bare minimum. Caring for someone with dementia well is an expensive business and the costs are increasingly borne by individuals and families.

The burden of dementia will not go away, indeed, being age-related, incidence will only increase with longer life expectancy. Unless funds and resources are increased dramatically the future for older people and their carers looks bleak.

Note

[1]   Thanks to Alzheimer's Society for permission to reproduce these extracts from articles first published in the Alzheimer's Disease Society newsletter in May 1994 and October 1994.

22

Cracks in the System

Pat Brown

My story echoes that of so many others who care for a young person with dementia: a story of misdiagnosis, misconceptions and lack of training in service providers. We kept coming up against the ageism within the system, which leads to many illogical situations, and which often prevents younger people with dementia from receiving appropriate care.

My husband Chris was a university lecturer, involved in the management of postgraduate programmes, consultancy work and research. We were married for 36 years, and he was an adoring father to our two daughters.

He was first diagnosed with anxiety and depression in 2000, when he was 50 years old. His father had died that year and work pressures had increased through restructuring, so this diagnosis seemed logical; anti-depressants were prescribed. We noticed that Chris seemed to have no interest in hobbies that had been important to him. He stopped playing golf, lost interest in photography, and stopped playing the piano. He had little concentration, and no longer read books or newspapers, all of which had been a large part of his life at the university. He found socialising difficult, even within family gatherings, and we also noticed his drinking of alcohol increased quite alarmingly.

In 2002 his mother died, and pressure at work continued to exhaust him. His anxiety worsened and we noticed he was getting more confused. He had difficulty making decisions, and signs of memory loss became evident. He also suffered numerous health problems, with his hip, his knee, his bladder and bowels, all of which were investigated thoroughly. But no physical cause could be found for any of the symptoms. I also noticed phobias – a desperate fear of heights and going out of the house. He would have severe panic attacks at the very mention of going out socially. He would go to the toilet constantly. He became obsessive and compulsive in his behaviour, adopting a regimental rigour to taking medication, and cleaning the kitchen compulsively. Life had to be a routine, and anything unexpected would cause confusion. He would check the content of his work briefcase time and time again before going to work, and his work diary became his bible. In November 2002, with his memory problems becoming more evident and his anxiety levels reaching new heights, he was advised by the doctor to take time off from work. Chris attended counselling sessions in the hope that 'talking therapy' might help him.

The GP continued to monitor Chris's condition and the anti-depressants were increased in strength. Chris was referred to a 'psychiatrist of the working age' within the mental health team in 2003. The psychiatrist supported the GP's diagnosis of stress, anxiety and depression, and the medication remained the same. Chris continued to attend counselling sessions, but only if I attended with him.

In February 2004, Chris was referred to a psychologist and underwent four hours of testing. His anxiety levels were high and his confusion was evident. He was unable to find the room after coming out for a break during the testing period. We waited until June for a follow-up appointment with the psychologist and the psychiatrist, and then found them apparently unwilling to believe the results of their own tests. The psychologist said that the results were inconclusive, but 'if Chris was as bad as the results showed, then he wouldn't be able to find the bathroom if he got up in the night, and he certainly wouldn't be able to drive through France on holiday'. He also said that, 'if the results were analysed by a neurologist he would have to surrender his driving licence'. I enquired as to whether they would support an application for Chris to take early retirement on health grounds, as his ability to function in the workplace seemed less and less likely, but they felt they were unable to support an application at this time and suggested that Chris return to work on a reduced timetable.

Consequently, Chris returned to work in July 2004, but as the start of the academic year approached, with the prospect of teaching, Chris became more anxious, more confused and greatly stressed. Inevitably, he was signed off again from work in September 2004, and an application for early retirement on health grounds was submitted. However, we did not include the report from the psychologist, who had concluded by commenting that Chris was obviously 'putting it on' in order to gain early retirement from his profession!

I was given a sabbatical from my college in 2005, on compassionate grounds, believing that I could give greater support to Chris if I was not working, and I could aid his recovery by providing mental stimulation. But his symptoms of anxiety continued and his confusion increased. I found that he could no longer remember directions to very familiar places. He had little confidence, was unable to do the simplest of tasks, and was frightened to go out in case he wanted to go to the toilet. If we did manage to go to the supermarket he would visit the toilet twice before leaving the house, and then again as soon as we arrived, and then after every couple of aisles he would need to go again. It was at this time I noticed that his driving was becoming erratic; in order to spare his feelings I would find excuses for me to do the driving wherever we needed to go.

At the end of 2005, I contacted our local branch of Mind, the mental health charity, whose outreach support workers visited Chris each week for eight weeks in early 2006, carrying out a programme designed to help him with his confidence. They would take him out to do a small amount of shopping on his own, and track his ability to select the goods and then take them to the checkout to pay for them. But after a few weeks his ability to manage these tasks did not improve and his anxiety levels were leading him to an even greater level of confusion. This led them to believe that Chris's problem was not one of mental health but was very likely to be a dementing illness. The support worker recommended to Chris's psychiatrist that he should have a CAT scan. The psychiatrist agreed and Chris had the scan. Three months later the results of the scan were given to me on the phone. I was told that there were no signs of a tumour but they felt that Chris should be assessed for his memory loss, and a referral was made to the consultant psychiatrist for the elderly. In August 2006 – six years after his symptoms had first appeared – an Alzheimer's dementia was diagnosed and medication was adjusted.

After the diagnosis was given, our review appointments continued with the psychiatrist of the working age, as at this time Chris was only 56 years old. But when I asked for further clarification about the dementia from which Chris was suffering, the psychiatrist of the working age told me he was a mental health specialist, and not an expert in dementing illness. When I insisted on having a psychiatrist who was an expert in dementia, I was informed that the psychiatrist for the elderly was the expert in dementia but Chris would not come under his care until he was 65 years old! I found this incredible, so I contacted PALS (Patient Advisory and Liaison Service) at the hospital, I wrote to the Alzheimer's Society and I contacted my MP. Eventually the situation was resolved and the psychiatrist for the elderly was allocated to his case.

When Chris was first diagnosed, his mini mental state score was 19/30, but twelve months later it had fallen to 7/30. I will always wonder whether earlier diagnosis and appropriate medication would have stabilised this deterioration. The words of the psychologist echoed in my ears: not only could my husband not find the bathroom at night, he was now totally confused as to what the toilet was. In the bathroom we have a toilet, hand basin and bath, but Chris had no concept about the usage of any of them.

After diagnosis, a list of care agencies was forwarded from the local authority. By this time Chris was displaying delusional behaviour and his mood would change according to various triggers, but I presumed that care agencies must be familiar with the symptoms of Alzheimer's, particularly as they were accredited by the local authority. Carers from the first care agency to which I entrusted my husband were obviously sorely lacking in dementia training. On the third week of visiting, I dared to leave Chris for an hour with the carer. On my return I found the carer in a worse state than the cared-for. The carer was outside in the garden smoking a cigarette, whilst Chris was wandering around confused and frightened in the house. The carer was obviously very disturbed by my husband's delusional state.

When I contacted the second agency, I explained fully the nature of my husband's erratic behaviour. When the senior carer visited for an assessment, Chris became very disturbed, but instead of calming and reassuring Chris, she challenged some of the delusional speak and exacerbated the situation. She then left. Later on in the day I received a phone call from the owner of the agency who said he was unable to entrust any of his carers to look after Chris. Clearly, this was yet another case of lack of dementia training within care agencies.

I was beginning to understand that Chris was not the archetypal Alzheimer's sufferer: he was young, physically fit, and delusional – not old and frail.

My next assault was day centres. If I was unable to get care at home, maybe I could take Chris out of the home. But no, this was not possible as day centres and respite care homes were not licensed for those under 65. (In desperation I wrote yet again to the local MP for assistance, and with his help, and the support of the consultant, a day centre facility specifically for people under 65 was eventually made available, although too late for us.) It appeared that there was no provision whatsoever within the whole of Bedfordshire for the younger person with dementia, but with the help of CSCI (the Commission for Social Care Inspection) I eventually found an agency based in Hertfordshire which was willing to service the Luton area where we live. They clearly recognised the issues of young people with dementia and trained their carers accordingly. They were able to engage Chris in activities around the house and garden; they understood the delusional nature of Alzheimer's, and together we discussed the triggers. The agency welcomed my involvement and provided me with techniques which would help me cope with an ever-changing condition.

Unfortunately, by the time that I had found the relevant service and the quality of care which met my husband's needs, the stabilisation that the medication was providing began to fail him. We did manage to celebrate Chris's fifty-seventh birthday in style, and his party was attended by all of his family and those friends who had remained steadfast in their support during his illness. The weather was beautiful and Chris was relatively well and happy with the day. But within the next month the deterioration was fast and furious.

He became more restless, his conversation was limited, his speech disjointed and his behaviour sometimes inappropriate. His delusions were becoming more frequent and more alarming. He would believe that there were people in the house; he would accuse me of killing his family or stealing his money. He became more aggressive verbally, with specific triggers such as taking a bath and getting undressed ready for bed. Delusions of men watching him naked were common, and there would be a barrage of abuse and threats. Once out of the bath, or in the bed, he would be calm and gentle again, with no memory of the experience. Driving with Chris became absolutely terrifying, as he would take off his seatbelt and attempt to get out of the car. He had no idea where he was, where we were going or indeed who I was, and he would threaten to kill me as he believed I was threatening his family. I learned very early never to challenge him. In order to defuse such a situation,

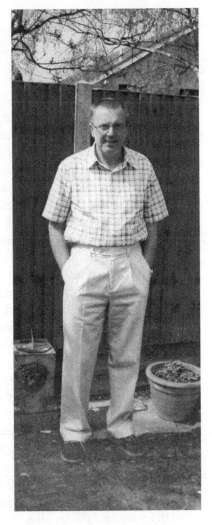

Chris Brown, spring 2007

I would speak softly and calmly, repeating over and over that I was his best friend and I would never hurt him.

Verbal aggression suddenly changed to physical aggression in August 2007. Initially this was directed to the carer, and then towards myself and the social worker. This triggered a chain of events that were emotionally devastating.

In an Alzheimer's sufferer, sudden physical aggression for no discernible reason can indicate the presence of an infection. We were therefore advised that he should attend the hospital's assessment centre so as to undergo investigations. Although Chris attended the centre, he was reluctant to stay and wanted to go home; sectioning under the Mental Health Act became inevitable.

Alzheimer's disease affords little dignity for the sufferer, but those providing support are expected to comply with high standards of dignified care. However, the process of sectioning lacks any semblance of dignity. Those in attendance are anonymous strangers, who instil fear and dread into the mind of the patient. Two doctors are in attendance, unfamiliar to both the carer and cared-for, along with uniformed police whose presence heightens fear, and an anonymous 'approved' social worker, whose role is a mystery. The doctors disappear after questions are asked and their duties done, the social worker overwhelms you with the legalities of the process and the police presence is threatening. The severity of the situation and the consequences that follow are alarming. All the time, you attempt to calm and reassure a very confused, anxious and frightened Alzheimer's sufferer, hoping that a degree of dignity can exist. When the ambulance was delayed, the social worker asked if Chris would mind going in the police car, in handcuffs! No sense of dignity there then! The assessment unit deemed most suitable by the approved social worker was a unit of the working age. The client group were young people with mental health problems, many of them through drug and substance abuse, others with eating disorders, attempted suicides, and manic depressives. This was a volatile unit, totally unsuitable for a dementia sufferer. All the triggers for aggressive behaviour existed in the environment in which Chris now found himself. The social worker showed Chris and me his room and the location of the bathroom. She had no concept of his confusion and lack of understanding. When I pointed out that Chris would never be able to find the bathroom without support, she said it would be okay if Chris just 'peed on the floor'. So this is the dignity afforded by the service providers.

After numerous phone calls, badgering and pestering, I managed to secure a transfer to the assessment unit for the elderly, where dementia patients were specifically cared for.

Once in a more suitable environment, Chris still took time to settle. His medication was assessed and staff took time to get to know him. He was treated with the utmost dignity, gentleness, compassion and understanding. Although his condition deteriorated, I believe this was a consequence of the disease and not the side-effects of the medication he was given. His aggression reduced, and gradually his sleep pattern regained some order.

I spent my days predominantly on the unit, walking the corridors with Chris and entering his world. The staff supported and comforted me, and

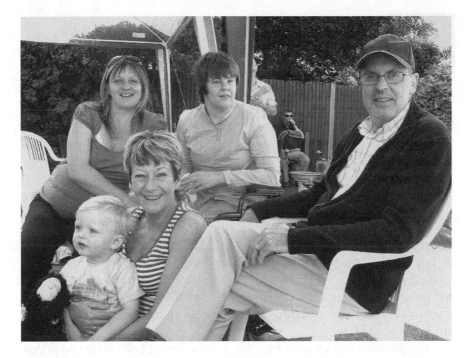

Chris and Pat with daughters Natalie (left) and Shelley, and grandson Joseph, July 2007

drip-fed me information on a need-to-know basis. I understood the disease and the inevitable consequence for the sufferer.

Chris was on the ward for three months before he was transferred to a nursing home. By that time he was doubly incontinent, and had suffered chest infections and pressure sores. He now had to be fed, and his appetite was waning; he suffered considerable weight loss. His periods of insight were now minimal, but on the limited occasions they occurred this was heaven-sent to me as the primary carer.

Chris was admitted to the nursing home on 14 December 2007. He was restless at first, but appeared to settle into his new environment well. He particularly enjoyed the gardens, not having experienced the outdoors for the previous three months. He would wander outside and feel the grass and the leaves on the trees. Maybe this was the beginnings of the infection that killed him, but the enjoyment the gardens gave him was uplifting. Unfortunately his body was too weak to fight the infection and he died on 26 December 2007, surrounded by his loving family.

23

Strained to the Limit

Andra Houchen

In July 2002, I sought counselling at my local GP practice. We had been leading a strange life, with my husband Anthony's inexplicable personality and behaviour problems, attributed to stress and depression by our GP and a psychiatrist. I had such a feeling of helplessness and hopelessness. I just did not know what to do.

The practice counsellor told me that I was a carer. I had no idea what this meant. As far as I knew I was a wife, a mother, going out to work, trying to help my husband who was ill in some unfathomable way, and doing my best to help him through this depression, bad patch or mid-life crisis.

Here is my record of Anthony's illness up to the point when he had to be admitted to hospital, showing how his dementia gradually and inexorably took over our lives.

December 2000

Illness begins to manifest as headaches, stomach aches, stress.

July 2001

Mr H is told he has depression; GP prescribes anti-depressant. Mr H thinks that there is something going wrong in his head and asks the GP why he isn't 'thinking properly'. GP says it is connected to the depression and stress.

Mr H has trouble remembering if he's done things, keeps checking whether he is doing the right things with rest of family, is obsessed with money, does not want to be alone, inflexible about mealtimes, leaves front door open when leaving house, has couple of incidents with car, wants to be with Mrs H all of the time.

September 2001

GP refers Mr H to private psychiatrist, Dr A. GP says 'Carry on taking tablets; carry on going to see Dr A.'

Mr H thinks he is getting better. Family notice that misunderstandings and cognitive mishaps increase but are always explained as 'one-offs' by Mr H.

Mr H repeatedly misjudges situations when driving: there is nearly a major accident when he accelerates instead of braking. Mrs H is terrified by this incident and bewildered that Mr H is totally unaffected by any thought that there was anything wrong with his driving. Mrs H pretends that there is something radically wrong with the car and gets rid of it. Even more puzzling that Mr H does not seem to care.

December 2001

Dr A diagnoses agitated depression and compulsive/obsessive disorder, but says he will not carry on treating Mr H due to his demands and repetitive behaviour – constant telephoning of office demanding to see him.

Mrs H accompanies Mr H to appointment with Dr A, and is left angry and upset at the result. Dr A treats Mr H as if he is stupid, and tells him that he must pull himself together and get out of his current state. Mr H does not understand how he can get out of his state: he is taking the tablets he has been told to take, and thinks he does feel a bit better. Mrs H leaves the appointment physically shaking and cries on the tube back into London. Mr H says he is the one that is ill and has no idea why Mrs H appears to be in a 'bad mood'. This makes Mrs H even more upset.

Mr H tells younger daughter (aged nineteen) that she will have to pay her university fees (£1,000) because he can't find the money. Mrs H has to smooth things over and produce the money.

Mrs H has instinctive feeling that depression is not the problem. She goes back to the GP with Mr H, and asks for an assessment for Mr H from the local NHS mental health team. Mr H says there is nothing the matter with him and he feels that Mrs H should see the mental health team.

GP tells Mr H to carry on taking the tablets; it's just depression, nothing more. Mr H must stop being a nuisance to the health service and the doctor's surgery; perhaps another tablet should be considered; these anti-depressants do take time to work. Mr H feels confident that taking the drugs will improve his state of mind.

Mrs H at wits' end, requests own referral for mental health. Mr H says he doesn't know why she can't cope and there is nothing wrong with the way he is behaving.

January 2002

Mrs H has mental health assessment and is told that because her problems are being caused by an external source (i.e. Mr H), and she does not have a mental illness, she will not be referred on to the mental health services. The assessment nurse agrees to see Mr H, although Mrs H is told this is highly irregular: the mental health team should not see both spouses from a marriage; this is not correct procedure.

Husband sees mental health assessment nurse and is referred to consultant psychiatrist at psychiatric hospital.

March 2002

Mr H starts seeing psychiatrist, Dr B. Mrs H goes with him every time, as an observer, not a contributor. Mr H also referred for psychological testing; Mrs H told not necessary to accompany Mr H for these tests.

May 2002

Mrs H becoming more desperate: after two visits to Dr B, continuation of same anti-depressants, nothing has changed at home. Mr H convinces Dr B that he is perfectly well apart from anxiety and depression. In reality, at home no one is allowed to make any noise, have any conversation, interfere in any way with Mr H's sleep pattern, etc. Meals must be taken when Mr H wants them, and there can be no radio, TV, telephone conversations, etc. if Mr H doesn't want them. Mr H wants to go to bed at 8.30 or 9 p.m. and then does not want to be disturbed till morning. Mrs H has to creep around in the evening; Mr H does not want her to go out as he doesn't want to be alone. Relationships at home are strained to the limit.

Eventually Mrs H tells Dr B that what Mr H is saying (i.e. that he is not causing any disruption to home life) is not true. Mrs H has to tell Dr B these things in front of Mr H. Mr H becomes aggressive towards Mrs H as he cannot understand that there is anything abnormal in his behaviour. Dr B presents an icy front and advises that Mr H must continue to take the anti-depressants as they must be given time to work. No help or explanation or advice is offered to Mrs H.

Mrs H and daughters cannot do anything right. Mr H insists on accompanying Mrs H to work every day and then goes back home on his own to work. As soon as he gets home he starts telephoning Mrs H and carries on phoning her all day. Wants to know exactly when she will be back, what he should eat for lunch, who he should phone in his business. Mr H starts walking round the house naked when getting up and going to bed – daughters are badly affected by this sight. Finances are strained but husband keeps saying finances are fine; says he has lots of work coming on stream, shows Mrs H a bona-fide-looking work plan. Plan seems perfectly logical and reasonable. (How wrong can one be!)

July–October 2002

Mr H's symptoms worsen.

Anthony was taken into hospital for assessment in November 2002. I still had no diagnosis for him except anxiety and agitated depression. When he went into hospital, my own state of mind was muddled and confused, and emotionally I felt a mess. I had already had over a year of strange behaviour that neither I nor the rest of the family could understand. We had somehow just kept limping along. Because he hadn't been sectioned, he suddenly reappeared

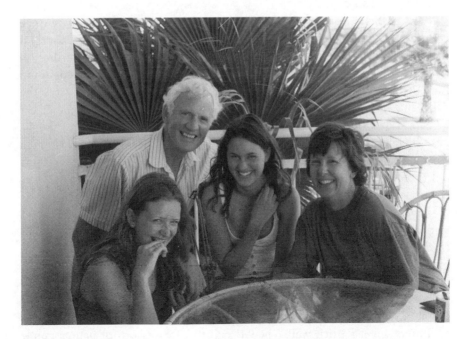

Anthony and Andra Houchen with daughters Louisa (left) and Amanda, 1997

after a couple of days, and although I eventually managed to get him back to the hospital, he was obviously very angry with me and shouted at me and pushed me away when we got back there. This was deeply wounding. I felt incapable of doing anything – even talking about what was happening. I went home and dissolved into a heap of tears and woe. Fortunately, a good friend came and put me to bed for a couple of days in her house, and that enabled me to have a bit of rest and then to go home again. As most of us do, I found some inner strength from somewhere to carry on.

Anthony was having his own problems, trying to understand his strange new world in a psychiatric hospital and coping with his fellow patients who had a range of acute psychiatric conditions. I went to the doctor to explain that I felt near collapsing myself and he prescribed sleeping tablets. I badly needed to talk to someone who knew and understood what I was going through, but there was no one.

My employer gave me two weeks' sick leave to sort myself out and it was then that I started looking through Anthony's finances. I was appalled by what I discovered, sick with worry at the enormity of financial muddle that he had created. He had made misjudgements in his business and had taken out two bank loans and five credit cards; there were thousands of pounds of debt. Overnight, I had to turn my hand to financial fire-fighting and try to put out as many fires as I could.

The financial institutions deal entirely differently with debts where there is a diagnosis of brain disease or dementia rather than a diagnosis of a mental illness such as depression. It was not until one and a half years further on that I had a definite diagnosis of dementia. Only then could I get recognition from the financial institutions that my husband would not be able to settle the debts that he had incurred, as he would not be able to work again, and that he had made financial misjudgements due to brain disease and not mental illness. In any case, he had no money to pay back what he owed. Many of these companies hounded me to pay my husband's debts, and again it was some time before I realised that much as I wanted to pay all this money back, I was not responsible for paying it out of my own pocket. Once I had the diagnosis of dementia, I was able to either get the debt written off or come to arrangements with the banks and finance companies. The only nut that I couldn't crack was the Inland Revenue, who were adamant that my husband had to pay his tax bill in full. However, they did agree that I could pay the money in instalments, which they said was a huge concession on their part.

During the first year of my husband's illness, I had tried to talk to our GP about how life was becoming odd and strange for myself and our two daughters. I met a brick wall. The GP said that for reasons of patient confidentiality he could not discuss anything about my husband with me. We had been with the GP practice for around eighteen years, and with this GP for about eight years. I could go to an appointment with my husband, but only as an onlooker, and there could be no separate discussion with me concerning my husband's case. It appeared that nothing I said would be taken into account, despite the GP's knowledge of us as a family: we had no history of depression or stress or nervous breakdown or marital problems. But my husband was being perceived and treated as if he were a single person, with no consideration given to the other three people in the family. During the long wait for the diagnosis, we had to live with inexplicable personality and character changes unaided, because Anthony was adamant that there was nothing wrong with him.

I was completely ignorant myself in matters of both mental health and brain disease, so I relied on what my GP said and what the consultant psychiatrist in the acute psychiatric section of our local hospital said. In the heart of London, you might think the very best advice and resources would be available to recognise that there was a lot more going wrong with my husband than anxiety and depression – but sadly this was not the case. Because this type of dementia is unusual, it may only be seen once or twice in a GP's career, if at all. The psychiatrists we saw seemed equally unaware of this particular condition.

Anthony was in and out of the psychiatric hospital for a year and given a variety of anti-depressants and ECT (electro-convulsive therapy). My daughters and I were not happy with ECT being administered to Anthony, but in the face of the recommendations of two professionals who advised this treatment we reluctantly agreed.

It was not until October 2003 that the word dementia was finally mentioned. References had been made to an organic or physical cause of Anthony's illness, but in my ignorance I had not linked this to dementia. As soon as he was over 65, the consultant at the psychiatric hospital moved him out, into the care of a psychogeriatric unit in another hospital. The consultant of the other hospital did at least know of fronto-temporal dementia and Pick's disease and spent some time with Anthony and me explaining about dementia. To Anthony it had about as much meaning as telling someone they have a common cold. He was quite pleased to know that he had something called Pick's disease and that he did not have depression. I knew as the consultant was talking that I was not actually understanding the words. It was several months before I could really get to grips with what the effects of this would be on Anthony, myself and our two daughters. There was no one to talk to who could give us emotional support, or help in practical ways, and we felt very much alone. I still had to carry on working, and I still had the constant worry of sorting out the thousands of pounds of debt that Anthony had amassed.

In January 2004, the diagnosis was confirmed by the National Hospital for Neurology and Neurosurgery in London. Pressure was put on me to find an EMI (elderly mentally infirm) home and move Anthony out of the hospital he was in.

After searching and searching for anything which seemed remotely suitable that was near enough to London, I found a place in Sussex in May 2004. Although the facilities were not out of the ordinary, the manager of the home had experience of caring for another person with fronto-temporal dementia, and so we moved Anthony there. However, although they were doing their best, it was soon obvious that the nursing home could not in fact meet his needs. I gave up my London job and rented a flat near to Anthony, and I supplement his care most days of the week, except for the days I work. As a result of what has happened to us, I have trained in dementia care as a job. I now work two days a week running day centres for people who have been affected by dementia; one of the days is specifically for people affected at an early age.

This tale is still not at an end, as the manager of the home now says that he can no longer look after Anthony even with all my support. We are now looking at alternative homes together, and I hope that this time we will finally be able to get Anthony the care that he deserves.

Break on Through to the Other Side

Louisa Houchen

One of the strangest and hardest things to deal with is to grieve for your father whilst he's still alive, and that's what I went through when my dad, Anthony, first developed Pick's disease – and lost his personality along with it. People would say that he was still alive and physically fit, so why had I crumbled into a shadow of my former self? At that time, I suffered from chronic insomnia. I would go to bed and all I could think about was the confusion that we felt as a family. A diagnosis was not made for a long while; there were no answers.

Visits to the hospital in London when he first became ill were hellish. Everything about that place and how he was treated was horrific. For example, he was given electric shock treatment, and was kept in a basement, sharing a very cramped room with some small high windows with other 'inmates', whilst essential building work was carried out. My sister and I would cry and he couldn't understand what 'the wet thing' was on our faces. His quality of life there was very poor. There was no one to watch over him properly, and he was allowed to 'go for a walk' on his own. This was extremely dangerous as he could have been injured or worse, and was very upsetting for me, as I worked nearby and would see him wandering the streets alone in my lunch break; then I would go back to work and feel unable to talk to anyone.

I think of those days as the 'dark days' and I have more or less blotted them out now. Sometimes I feel as though three years of my life went missing down a black hole, but at other times I realise I just needed to be upset and to deal with thoughts and feelings, before I could come out the other side. Through exercise and meditation I learnt to be happy again, and by the time I was in my late twenties I was almost back to 'normal'.

I never really felt I could speak to my friends about my father and how I was dealing with it, but I talked at great length about things with my sister.

One morning, I found myself walking to the doctor's surgery to speak with a counsellor. This helped me to realise that I didn't have a problem with myself, and that it was time to let go of feeling as though I had fallen apart and start to enjoy my life again. I reminded myself that that's what my dad would have wanted.

My sister and I both found that a song by The Doors kept running through our minds. It goes, 'Break on through to the other side', and that's what I think we've both managed to do.

Thank goodness my mother is an amazing person who helps to care for him and who has put much effort into her own research as to how he can be looked after and how to secure funds for this. There still seems to be a very 'Victorian' view of how to deal with people who suffer from brain disease: it is shrouded in mystery, kept locked away and never discussed. Brain disease should be brought out into the open, and sensible solutions should be thought of. A positive attitude must prevail in order for things to improve.

25

Rocking the Boat

Sheena Sanderson

'I know! You're not trying to take over the world with the Millennium Bug. It's killer bees!' This was my 49-year-old husband accusing me of yet another wild plot.

Philip was diagnosed with Parkinson's disease at the age of 32. We'd met when he was working as a university lecturer and I was departmental secretary and we'd got together over the Guardian crossword. Philip was a quiet, intellectual man who loved walking, cooking and photography – and me. We were very much in love, and we left our respective marriages and started living together, getting married in 1980. He already had symptoms then, but the GP said he was 'attention-seeking' and prescribed tranquillisers.

For the first five years after diagnosis he was able to work. By then he was a senior IT consultant with an oil company, but he had to retire at the age of 37. Over the years the illness changed and he developed very severe involuntary movements, leading people to think he was drunk or mentally disabled. At the age of 40, I became his main carer, full-time, for the princely sum of £41.41 per week, while he took more and more pills and injections to control the illness. In 1996 he fell and broke his shoulder, although this wasn't diagnosed for two years. By this time his involuntary movements were so violent that they would literally throw him off the bed.

Finally, a surgeon agreed to fit a replacement shoulder, but brain surgery was needed to stop the movements on one side. He came home in a euphoric mood, talking about getting his driving licence back, buying a motorbike: very scary for me. I could see that he had no idea of his condition: he was like a clockwork toy winding down in front of my eyes. He finally realised he wasn't 'cured', said, 'I saw Heaven!' and burst into tears.

Then he went into a phase where nothing was ever right: no clothes comfortable, the house was too hot/too cold, and he was having hallucinations.

He came out with all sorts of theories that were completely mad. He accused me of anything he could think of and became very nasty. He told his social worker that I was abusing him by turning the heating off, not feeding him and hitting him regularly. Although this could easily have been disproved by the agency carers who came twice a day, I was on the verge of being branded a criminal by having a Vulnerable Adult Protection procedure placed on me, which could have involved the police and could have stopped me seeing him.

The Parkinson's Disease Society information states that people with Parkinson's often go on to develop dementia, but this is played down in order not to worry sufferers. Because Philip was labelled 'disabled' by social services, and there was nothing in his records indicating mental deterioration, they assumed that he just had a *physical* disability and that his mind was normal. When you have social services involved, they *have* to believe the 'service user', that is, him not me. There seems to be no leeway in this because they have a policy which is followed in all circumstances even when it defies common sense.

The mental health manager who came to assess him when he was talking about 'killer bees' (I was going to stun them, attach bombs to their legs and put about 20,000 in a box and send them to enemy territories) said he found no sign of mental problems and that he thought it was 'emotional and financial abuse' on my part! (I have since managed to get the medical records changed and received a full apology. The manager no longer works there, but this shows how easy it is to be accused of abuse and not even know it.)

We had constant battles with the authorities over the years, mainly because his condition was unusual and he seemed to slip through the net. At this point, he was attending a council day centre twice a week to give me a break. This was a frightening time for me. Philip felt that the devil was controlling him and he 'saw' things on the walls that weren't there. He constantly looked for cameras which he thought were filming him and thought all the staff were foreign as he couldn't understand them. I later found out that the staff were very sceptical when I mentioned his delusions, as he had only expressed these thoughts to me. Someone there actually called a solicitor to advise him on divorce! I knew nothing of this until much later when he was in hospital and the bill mysteriously appeared by his bed.

He was admitted to a neuro-behavioural unit where he stayed for five months, and I was then told that he needed to be in a specialised care home. Then began another series of huge problems.

The first home was specifically for brain-damaged younger people and I naively didn't realise that many of the patients had learning disabilities. While he was there, the home was inspected by CSCI (the Commission for Social Care Inspection) who advised me to make a complaint to them about his lack of care. When I did this, the matron retaliated by giving him notice to leave! You then have one month in which to find somewhere a) that takes 'younger' people, that is, those under 60, b) that has a vacancy and c) that you trust.

On the social worker's advice, he moved to a home nearer my house. I had misgivings as he'd been in this home for respite in the past, but I had no knowledge of my rights and acted on the information given. This was a big mistake! Philip was neglected: he developed blisters on his thighs, which were left untreated for nine months, and eventually developed MRSA. They didn't bother to clean his teeth, and he had to have seven of them out under general anaesthetic. I later found out that his evening meal was being whisked away because he was tired and couldn't feed himself. CSCI could do nothing unless I made a complaint; as soon as I did, they immediately investigated. The matron was so angry that she accused me of psychologically abusing him and I was put through the Vulnerable Adult Protection procedure unsupported. I lost two weeks of my life, spending over six hours on the phone to the Samaritans during that period before being found innocent.

Social services did nothing to help me, quite the reverse, because they had other clients in the home and didn't want to rock the boat. Obviously, I wanted to move him after what I'd been through, but I was told I couldn't as 'his needs were being met'!

Just at this time, his care was taken over by the primary care trust (PCT), much to my relief, as I had found social services extremely unhelpful. I quickly found another home locally where I was promised wonderful care. Unfortunately, Philip was dumped in a corner in a room full of people with Alzheimer's and didn't understand what was going on. One day, he managed to get up and walk through two rooms, up a flight of stairs and along a corridor to get to his own room. The matron said she couldn't take responsibility for him and asked us to move him!

By now, I'd had enough, and asked the PCT to help by admitting Philip to the local community hospital where I could visit every day until we found somewhere suitable where we wouldn't be let down again. Ha ha!

So he then went to the fourth home, which I was assured gave excellent care. But, very quickly, things started to deteriorate.

I went to visit Philip just before Christmas and found a few things wrong. I'd always rung the PCT staff to check I wasn't overreacting, so this is what I did. The nurse assessor asked me if certain things agreed at the last meeting had happened, and they hadn't, so she rang the matron. A few minutes later the matron came storming in and started yelling at me: I tried to calm her down and Philip got upset and started crying.

By the time I'd left and driven to a local car park to ring the PCT, she'd given Philip notice. Immediately I rang CSCI, who said it was a serious matter, but they took months to investigate, and it all got watered down.

By now, I was beginning to think that I'd never find anywhere suitable. I rang the CSCI inspector who'd helped me at the second home; she was now an area manager for a chain of care homes. She told me there was a room vacant in one of them and I was totally confident that with her in charge, everything would be fine. It was, until she was suddenly made redundant without any warning!

Things were deteriorating again, but when I tried to move Philip, the PCT said I couldn't as 'his care needs were being met', so I had a major battle on my hands. In the end I had to make a formal complaint to the home, which upset a lot of people, before I was finally allowed to move him. The present home is the only one I've been able to visit and look round myself without any pressure.

This is the sixth home in seven years and I've had to battle with the council, the Local Government Ombudsman, the Health Service Ombudsman, Nursing and Midwifery Council, the Commission for Social Care Inspection, the local PCT and now the Healthcare Commission. It seems to me that there is no one taking responsibility for the running of care homes and everyone passes the buck.

Philip is now happy. He spends most of his time laughing, usually at totally inappropriate things, and has become very childlike in a lot of ways. He's now institutionalised and can do very little himself. It still breaks my heart to see him like this, but after seven years it gets easier.

So now my husband, who has a first class honours degree in economics and a master's degree, has become a person who no longer walks, is totally incontinent and hardly able to communicate. As the years go by, it seems that it's only me who remembers him as he was when we got married.

At first he was very frightened and I spent ages reassuring him that everything was all right and that he wasn't going to be evicted and homeless. Now he seems less worried and his face lights up when he sees me. Last year, he even asked me to marry him! He has private physiotherapy and massage/reflexology twice a week, which I'm sure are helping his posture and communication.

Philip hasn't lived at home now for over seven years, and I have another man in my life. I feel I've earned a bit of happiness and normality but find that some people have stopped speaking to me: these are people who never visited us when Philip was at home and never even tried to imagine what my life was like. It hurt me at first, but I'm proud that I have done whatever I can, and still keep doing it, to make sure my husband is as well looked after as possible.[1]

Note

[1] Philip died in March 2009. Names have been changed.

26

The Significant Other

Brian Baylis

Timothy was a gay man suffering from an extreme form of dementia and a number of other life-threatening illnesses.

We were not partners, but like many other gay men, we had a very close and affectionate friendship. Such friendships, particularly in a situation of dementia, are as significant as partnerships, and the role of the 'significant other' in the whole process of care needs to be acknowledged. At the time of his death, aged 65, after nearly ten years of severe illness, we had known each other for 40 years.

Timothy's dementia came upon him suddenly, and he was at first placed in the large general psychiatric ward of a run-down mental hospital. A year or so later, after my intervention, he went to live in a small care home for residents with differing kinds of mental disability, where he stayed for eight years. When the care home closed, he was relocated to a nursing home for severely mentally disabled people for a further year and then spent the last year of his life in continuing care at a mental hospital.

His next of kin lived in Ireland, and made little contact with social services for the first eight years. There were few visits. Social services referred to me as Timothy's advocate and carer, and involved me in all meetings and matters relating to his medical, psychological and general care. I visited Timothy at least three times a week, and regularly took him out.

When Timothy first came into care, he was totally confused, with almost no short-term memory and only small fragments of long-term memory. He had chronic liver failure and diabetes. He was also agitated, very unhappy and at times aggressive as a result of his fears, condition and circumstances. His sister came across from Ireland in the early days of his illness, with a view to having him transferred to Ireland, and taking powers of attorney. After a considerable delay, she decided to do neither of these things and Timothy became a ward of court.

Timothy seemed a sad and hopeless case to hospital staff, but I had a strong feeling that his quality of life could be improved, and was determined to do everything I could to make this happen.

With the encouragement of the social worker and the psychiatrist, I began taking Timothy out in my car, on visits to places in Hampstead, where he had lived for 30 years or so. We walked on the Heath and visited Highgate Ponds, and he developed a great tenderness for the various water fowl. Weekly visits to my home on a Saturday were another important part of Timothy's life. He loved to view the garden from the conservatory, to cook meals together and to help prune bushes and shrubs in the garden.

I also began taking him out to pubs for meals. Timothy had previously had drink problems, and there was some anxiety that he would crave alcoholic drinks in a pub setting. However, he was happy to drink alcohol-free lager, not realising that there was no alcohol in it. In particular, I took Timothy to a gay pub in Hampstead he knew well. I explained Timothy's problems to the bar staff, and a quiet corner table was kept for us. Little by little, Timothy re-learned how to play a simple game of dominoes. His concentration, and the joy he derived from this, were moving to witness. The bar staff and some of the 'regulars' were extremely kind. They came across when I nodded to them and had brief conversations – which were almost always the same, many hundreds of times over, throughout the years, without Timothy realising it. He never learned to recognise any of them, but this did not diminish the joy he experienced from these brief conversations in a familiar setting.

He plainly did not belong in hospital, and I pressed for some time for him to be moved to a care home. Eventually, the psychiatrist organised this. I arranged for the purchase of a TV and video from his funds, for use in Timothy's room, where he had to spend a great deal of his time. He had always had an interest in films, and had been a keen dancer as a young man, so I began showing him bits of films like *West Side Story* and *The Sound of Music*. Over many hundreds of showings, he began to get the shape and sequence of the stories in his mind and take delight in the music, dance and drama. Sometimes he was able to anticipate the dialogue, guess the next musical number and sing the songs. There was a noticeable intensity and steadiness of attention, and the experiences temporarily rescued him from the succession of relatively unrelated impressions and events which made up most of his life.

I also arranged for him to attend an Alzheimer's day centre a couple of miles away. I cannot speak too highly of the kindness and care shown to Timothy by the staff there. They became friends and advocates at the review meetings and elsewhere and made a very important contribution to Timothy's life over the years.

In general, Timothy's placement at the care home was fortunate. It took him some years to become familiar with the layout of the house, to find his way to the toilet and to his room, and also to feel some degree of comfort with the staff and the small number of other residents. It also took the staff some time to become familiar with Timothy's mood changes and frustrations, and to be able to deal effectively with these.

It was thought necessary, particularly in the early days, for Timothy to spend a great deal of his time in his room. Early on this worked reasonably well, as his room-mate did not need to be there apart from during sleeping hours. But when this resident died, the needs of the new resident – who wanted to spend lots of time in the room 'reading' devotional books – clashed with those of Timothy. As Timothy's almost entire stimulus related to watching and listening to TV and videos, it posed a big problem. It was depressing to observe Timothy, who was somewhat deaf, trying to follow video films for hours on end with barely audible sound. I was repeatedly told about the increase in Timothy's aggression and difficulties in managing him. I had to point out that I thought the two problems were linked. When I visited, I was also encountering Timothy in an even more confused and dopey state, which I considered to be due to altered medication.

Things got so bad that Timothy was removed to a general psychiatric ward in hospital where he immediately became severely disorientated and covered in a psoriatic rash – and was crouched up like a frightened animal. I was visiting him each day, speaking with the staff, and eventually was invited to a meeting at the hospital, chaired by the consultant, with the manager of the care home and all the medical specialists who had observed and assessed Timothy since his admission into hospital. Timothy's social worker – referred to as a 'key player' – did not turn up, but I was able to speak to the meeting, and there was very helpful input from medical staff, so that Timothy was re-admitted to the care home after about ten days. Things became better when, after much campaigning on my part, Timothy was given his own room.

I was fearful and concerned when the council decided to close the care home where Timothy was living. He was relocated to a nursing home for the severely mentally disabled, and although it was far from easy, the staff worked hard to help Timothy adjust to his new surroundings. I had regular meetings with the manager, as well as attending the review meetings and monthly in-house carers' meetings. However, he no longer received the monthly psychiatric input which he used to get, and I believe that he was being given increasingly large doses of risperidone, whereas at the previous care home it had been administered very sparingly. He became very lethargic, and more confused than before; his speech became increasingly slurred. Also, for the first time, he became doubly incontinent. After six months in the nursing home, he was admitted to hospital for investigation, but he continued to decline until his death almost a year later. I firmly believe that he was suffering from risperidone poisoning.

While he was living in the nursing home, a representative of Timothy's family suddenly made contact with social services, and from then on, at the family's direction, I was excluded from participation in all aspects of Timothy's care – financial, medical and psychiatric. All that remained was for me to visit Timothy, which I did on average four times weekly, and, when things were bad, every day. To the end, I remained Timothy's only regular frequent visitor.

During this period, when Timothy was in and out of different hospitals in a desperate state, the staff refused to give me any details of his medical condition on my daily visits. The nursing staff were always very apologetic, and I think somewhat puzzled, but they were clearly acting under direction.

On one occasion when Timothy was admitted to hospital, I arrived there to be told it was not possible to see Timothy. My response was that I would sit out in the waiting area all night if necessary, until they changed their minds. After an hour or so, they did. When I came into the area in which Timothy had been placed, I found him totally disorientated, very fearful, and ranting in virtually unintelligible, slurred speech. He was being held down by two burly hospital auxiliaries to prevent him from leaving the bed. I told them quietly that there was no need for this now. At first they did not believe me, and were surprised that Timothy recognised me and that I was able to communicate with him, listening to what he was desperately trying to say, and repeating the thoughts he was trying to express. He quietened down, and the auxiliaries disappeared. Despite all of this, and the fact that I was the only person whom Timothy recognised and could communicate with, the staff were still unable to give me details of his condition. I believe that his difficulties were created largely as a result of the large dose of risperidone, which was now being withdrawn.

Subsequently, Timothy recovered a little and became somewhat quieter, and the decision was taken to place him in continuing care and transfer him to a hospital for severely mentally disabled people, where he remained until his death. I was forbidden to attend the meeting which admitted Timothy to continuing care, and indeed all future care meetings, despite the fact that the team leader and social worker did not consider that this was justified or in Timothy's interests. Given the situation, I believe that social services should have arranged a meeting with the consultant, medical and care staff, family representative, social worker and myself, to enable me to object publicly to the decision to exclude me after nine years of attending all the care and review meetings as Timothy's only representative, during which the family had never been involved.

Social services had acknowledged my role as Timothy's chief carer and advocate over the previous nine years, and I have seen internal correspondence which states there was no case to exclude me. Yet no one from social services supported me or attempted to exert some moral pressure on the family, and expose the absurdity of their attitude.

I was extremely concerned that by admitting Timothy into continuing care, they were removing all the familiar props which were so vital to his wellbeing. I wanted to warn them that by taking him away from familiar living surroundings and staff, discontinuing his attendance at the Alzheimer's day centre (which had been a part of his life for nine years), and withdrawing vital visits to familiar places, Timothy would become completely disorientated, and would not be able to come to terms with his new environment. My worries had been anticipated in a psychiatric report two years earlier.

As for 'continuity of care' – even my letters to social services requesting new glasses and dentures for Timothy were ignored. I was told eventually that Timothy was no longer the concern of the social service department, and I should address my concerns to the continuing care team. I wrote to the continuing care team leader, attempting to put Timothy's life situation into some kind of context, and explaining my role. The reply came that they were unable to discuss Timothy's personal details because of 'issues of confidentiality'.

I had taken Timothy for an eye test over a year previously, but despite various requests, had not been permitted by the social worker to purchase new spectacles. In the end I was told to submit the prescription to the family representative, who eventually sent through the post a pair of entirely unsuitable, very heavy spectacles which did not fit and just fell off Timothy's face.

Although Timothy was becoming more and more disorientated, he still recognised extracts from his favourite videos, and right to the end he was able to join in singing some of the songs. I think the staff were surprised that Timothy still had this degree of engagement. Yet suddenly, his five videos disappeared from his room. The family representative refused to buy any new copies out of Timothy's funds, claiming the ward staff were of the opinion that he didn't need them. When I asked the ward staff for their support, they were plainly embarrassed and did not wish to be involved. I then did the only thing possible, and bought copies myself, which Timothy and I continued to watch until two days before he died.

The final indignity came on the day of Timothy's death. I had been visiting each day for some time as he was very unwell, and I had stayed until about 10.30 p.m. the night before. It was thought he could last in his coma-tose state for a day or two longer. But at seven the next morning I was phoned by the ward staff to say that he had died. By the time I got to the hospital, his body had been removed from the hospital mortuary by the family who had also removed all his possessions from his room. When I contacted the family representative, she said that it would not be possible for me to visit Timothy's body or attend his funeral. This is an example of the ruthless determination of the family to exclude me in all possible ways.

When the family removed Timothy's possessions, they also removed enlargements of my own photographs, which I had placed around the walls of Timothy's room in an attempt to give him some visual reminder of things and people he remembered. I wrote to the family twice, asking for the return of these, and asking also if they would tell me where his ashes had been interred. There was no reply.

For well over a year before Timothy's death, I had been complaining to social services about their appalling, unjust and authoritarian treatment of Timothy and myself, and their failure to act in his best interests. Most of my letters were simply ignored, so I had begun pursuing a number of issues through the council's complaints procedure. The most important issue of all was my exclusion from Timothy's care and the impact this had on his wellbe-ing. I believe very strongly that the whole sequence of actions by the council, colluding with the family and removing me from Timothy's care, was unethi-cal and unprofessional. In excluding me, they were removing from the care process Timothy's closest friend, and the only person whom he recognised. I was the one and only person who could provide a link with past experience and ensure continuity of care – which social services and the NHS claim to be greatly concerned about.

I made no headway with my complaints to the council and, in the mean-time, Timothy died. I resolved to take matters to the Local Government Ombudsman, but I was delayed for a whole year because I did not receive the relevant documents from the council. The case with the Ombudsman lasted almost three years. He found that the council had not acted appropriately with regard to the 'significant other', and directed the council to rewrite two of their key policies, and to inform him of the ways in which they intended to disseminate and implement them. However, the Ombudsman failed to follow this up, and I had to pursue him. When he investigated, he found out what I already knew – that the new policies had not been implemented. The Ombudsman imposed upon the council, on two separate occasions, awards of damages to myself, which I have given to charity.

I believe it is vital that the recent Mental Capacity Act[1] is contextualised for LGBT (lesbian, gay, bisexual and transgender) people and that its basic principle, namely, that the interests of the patient are always paramount, is enshrined in all policies of councils and NHS Trusts. Recognising the vital role of the 'significant other' in all care matters is part of this. Short-circuiting this with arguments about confidentiality is totally unacceptable. Confidentiality must operate in the interests of patients and not against them.[2]

When gay men have 40 years of shared history, it is very special. I shall always regard my friendship with Timothy as one of those rare, transforming friendships. There was lots of joy, even in the depths of dementia. However, sadly, the horrors of watching a loved one tormented and falling apart with dementia will always be with me, as will the way we were treated by the family, and by the authorities whose duty it is to care for vulnerable people.[3]

Notes

[1] See Alzheimer's Society *Factsheet* 460: *The Mental Capacity Act 2005*. Available at www.alzheimers.org.uk/factsheet/460, accessed 27 March 2009.

[2] See CSCI (2008) *Putting People First: Equality and Diversity Matters 1: Providing Appropriate Services for Lesbian, Gay and Bisexual and Transgender People*. Available at www.cqc.org.uk/_db/_documents/putting_people_first_equality_and_diversity_matters_1.pdf, accessed 27 March 2009. Printed copies available free on request on 0870 240 7535.

[3] Some details have been changed.

An Instruction Manual for Keeping your Mind

Gail Chester

Rule 1: *Avoid being born into a family where your grandmother dies with Alzheimer's shortly before your third birthday, your mother does the same three days before your fortieth, and your aunt, the last female in the line before you, dies with the condition a dozen years later.*

As Rule 1 is not really within your control, move on to **Rules 2 and 3**: *Trust your own thinking* (but not all the time); and, *Don't believe everything you read in the papers.* That is to say, when looking after people with dementia, there are no rules. But there may be gentle guidelines, and a certain comfort in knowing that you are not alone if you worry that you may succumb to dementia at any moment, and that you are as great an expert as the so-called experts.

I found that my biggest issue in having all these relatives with Alzheimer's was not the actual caring for them while they were ill, as I was lucky to have good relationships with them while they were healthy. No, the worst of it has been dealing with all the feelings in the aftermath. Prominent among them has been the fear of getting Alzheimer's myself, or that my sister will get it before I do, and then I will have to care for her, too.

Actually, I am quite philosophical about that, because of **Rule 4**: *Guilt is a pointless waste of time.* Remember that you are doing your best in very difficult, under-resourced circumstances, and that you will do a much worse job of caring for your loved one if you sacrifice your own life to do it. Thus, as I value my sanity, I would not hesitate to encourage her to go into residential care, and I do not think she would mind. Interesting, though, that we have never discussed this.

I asked my sister what she thought should go in this article – how did she feel while Mum was ill, how does she feel looking back on it? 'I don't remember,' she replied, and burst into uproarious laughter. Jokes like this wear very thin after the hundredth repetition. But underlying them is a very serious issue for both of us – are we going to inherit it?

Usually, I have no trouble constructing my pieces into seamlessly flowing, logically argued narratives. But what we are talking about here is watching the certain disintegration of the mind, the definite loss of flowing narrative. So I am having difficulty getting it together seamlessly. Perhaps, given the topic, it does not matter if you notice the joins. Perhaps it is no coincidence that in the months since I agreed to write this article, I have been plagued with the anxieties I want to document.

When I was a teenager, my mother was in her fifties – the age at which her mother started showing signs of Alzheimer's. It may have been a coincidence, and it may have been the menopause, but for several years my mother went round in a heightened state of tension, which was not easy to live with. I am in my fifties now, and even though my mother's Alzheimer's didn't start until her late sixties, I find myself constantly checking my brain minutely for signs that all is well – or not.

Occasionally I hear myself talking so slowly, the uninflected dirge bores even me. I hear myself leaving gaps in my speech, as my turgid brain grasps ineffectually for the right word. The sentences I manage to string together are much less elegantly expressed than they used to be. I don't know if anybody else can tell the difference – I don't dare ask.

Even though I know there are half a dozen reasons why one's memory can lapse, the automatic feeling is that I must be developing Alzheimer's. The first time my memory went was when I dislocated my pelvis. I tried to carry on working normally as I lay in bed, rigid with pain, phone in one hand, notebook propped up on a cushion. My unconscious mind knew what the rest of my brain didn't: I had to *stop*. My osteopath told me that stress is a common reason for memory loss, and that if I rested, it would return to normal. After a few weeks, it did.

When I was pregnant, I had a severe attack of maternal amnesia. This time my memory didn't return to normal, ever, though after a few years most of it came back (until the menopause started a few years after that…).

I met a man recently who told me that his wife had been sent to a memory clinic to see why her memory had suddenly deteriorated. I was amazed. I didn't know such institutions existed. They certainly didn't a few years ago. I wonder if I should get myself referred?

Rule 5*: Remember that it's not only people who are worried about getting Alzheimer's who set themselves little tests.*

'Write everything down as soon as you think of it and make a note before you forget.' This is what you are told in every writing class. So that's all right then, it's not just me: everybody needs to make notes to capture that fugitive idea that seems so great on the tube, in the supermarket, at 4 a.m. when you can't sleep. Later you can sift, your tutor tells you.

But what if you can't sift any more? As her Alzheimer's developed, my aunt would make increasingly obscure lists on the back of envelopes, in the margin of newspapers, on paper serviettes, in an effort to keep control of her thoughts. I found hundreds of them when I was clearing her flat, heartbreaking reminders of the person she had been and wanted to remain.

As it happens, my partner is a geneticist, a sceptical, radical geneticist who runs a campaign around issues of human genetics. When we met, my mother's Alzheimer's was already moderately advanced, but even though her short- and medium-term memory had substantially departed, she knew who Dave was until not long before she died. As one of my friends said, 'She waited 37 years for you to bring home a nice Jewish boy, and you think she's going to forget?' The first time I took him to meet my parents, Mum sat opposite him at the dining table, waving at him and smiling. Every ten minutes she would point beamingly at her pride and joy – the antique china cabinet with the tea sets she had collected over the years – and say to Dave in a knowing voice, 'One day all that will be yours.'

So naturally, early in our relationship, conversation turned to the likelihood of me inheriting my mother's Alzheimer's – along with the china cabinet. In the late 1980s, Dave was completely dismissive of the idea that my family's history of Alzheimer's meant that I was likely to inherit it, as he claimed that the early onset variety was the only type that could be inherited. More recently, he has modified his position a bit, and now says it is quite likely that there are extra copies of the susceptibility gene in my family, but it is still not a foregone conclusion that I will get Alzheimer's, and in any case, so what?

Dave's default position is that I shouldn't assume that I'm going to inherit Alzheimer's, as – unlikely as it sounds – three close family members with the disease could still be individual sporadic cases. I am usually the optimist in our house, but on a day when I can't remember if I have taken my vitamin pills and have spent ten minutes looking for my glasses case, I worry at him: how can you be sure that Alzheimer's is not round the corner? Of course I can't be sure, he says, trying not to be grumpy, but you know that not all memory loss is Alzheimer's, you know you may not have the susceptibility gene, and even if you do, getting it isn't inevitable. It doesn't matter how many times he tells me, I can't make myself entirely believe that if I have the gene I won't succumb.

So would I be happier if I took the test to see if I have got the susceptibility gene? Why would I be? There is nothing I can do about it, apart from taking the normal precautions of eating healthily and taking more exercise, which I ought to be doing anyway. If I got a positive result, all I could do would be to worry and feel terrified, and I might not end up getting Alzheimer's anyway.

Rule 6: *Do not be surprised if you are sometimes unable to distinguish between a rational fear and an irrational urge to eat an awful lot of chocolate.*[1]

Notes

[1] Readers concerned about these issues are referred to Alzheimer's Society *Factsheet 450: Am I at Risk of Developing Dementia?* and *Factsheet 405: Genetics and Dementia.* All the Factsheets may be downloaded at www.alzheimers.org.uk/factsheets. Printed copies of the Factsheets are available on request from Xcalibre on 01753 535751.

KEEPING IN TOUCH, LETTING GO

*W*hen Words Fail

Barbara Pointon

It had been snowing. At the window, Malcolm exclaimed, 'Just look at that bobbin!' Bobbin? Pause for thought… Ah yes, robin! Malcolm, some four years after diagnosis with Alzheimer's, had reached the stage where he felt that words dropped into a black hole, and he often came up with a word that rhymed with the one he wanted. The result, however amusing, even poetic, grimly indicated that his use of language was beginning to slip. It hadn't always been like that.

Malcolm had a real flair for words. He wrote scripts for the announcers on BBC's Third Programme (now Radio 3), was an engaging teacher of music (whether with a class of six-year-olds or lecturing to students at Cambridge) and invented satirical sketches and songs for our local drama group. When Malcolm was diagnosed in 1991, at the age of 51, I felt that the bottom had dropped out of our world.

First to go was spelling, then writing, then reading. Three years into the illness, speech began to falter and, as well as using rhymes, Malcolm would conflate two words to form another one. One day he told me that dinner was 'in the stoven' – a mixture of stove and oven. Trying to make sense of it all certainly kept me on my toes! As time went on, if I asked him a question, I learned to leave time for him to think and frame a reply and not to jump into the silence with more explanations, which would only confuse him further. But the hardest point at this stage was dealing with friends who didn't realise that people with dementia can understand far more than they can say. I lost count of the number of dinner parties where people hardly addressed a single word to him. The damaging sense of social isolation can begin early.

About six years into the illness, Malcolm's speech descended into gobbledegook. I could only tell by the tone of it what he was trying to communicate, and I had to rely on other cues, such as facial expression or body

language. In my own verbal communication with Malcolm, I learned to use
very simple words in short sentences,
or ask questions which needed only
yes or no answers. Even that had its
pitfalls: Malcolm went on to say yes to
everything, because I guess he thought
that's what I wanted to hear. Eventually
he was reduced to mere vocalisations
and noises. It's just like how you or I
learned to speak, but in reverse. I vividly
remember one evening when Malcolm's
brother and I were playing a duet on the
piano and I was making loads of mistakes. Malcolm's sense of melody and
harmony must still have been intact,
because he gave us the biggest and
rudest raspberry I have ever heard.

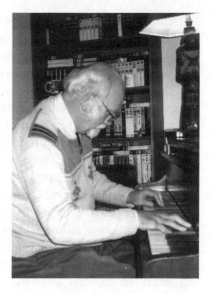

Malcolm Pointon, 1997

When words failed, it was music
that took over. Even though he was scoring zero on all the cognitive tests,
and intelligible speech was wholly gone, Malcolm could improvise for hours
on the piano. He could no longer remember pieces he once played, or indeed
read the music, and each piece was a new creation. Despite his normal memory
span being reduced to less than a minute, Malcolm would invent pieces where
he would set out musical ideas at the beginning and play them again near the
end, at least twenty minutes later. The improvisations also gave me a precious
insight into how he was feeling – happy, peaceful, angry, resigned or positive.
Many improvisations had a powerful, angry section, but most resolved into
an autumnal peace. I believe they were therapeutic for us both. Malcolm also
listened to recorded music (on a personal stereo with earphones to blot out
the rest of the world) and I sometimes chose recordings to alter his mood – to
calm frustration, or lift depression – rather than resorting to drugs. I stand in
awe of the power of music, because of its non-verbal nature, to get through
when other channels are blocked.

Some people seemed to think that Malcolm had become less of a person
once they couldn't have their normal kind of conversations with him, and took
some time to understand that communication isn't just about words; there are
other ways. In the late stage (which lasted seven years), after Malcolm became
mute and immobile, I had to gently remind careworkers who worked alongside me to carry on talking to Malcolm. We talk to babies who can't answer
back, don't we? The sound of the human voice is a very basic need.

Through my observation of Malcolm, I created a picture in my mind of how our sense of selfhood is built up – in a series of layers, a bit like an onion – and what happens when dementia takes a hold. We enter this world as a new baby, with an individual essence, identity, spirit, call it what you will, and this forms our central core. As a tiny baby, a second layer starts to form: we explore our surroundings using our five senses; we experience emotions and our psychological self begins to develop. Then, as a small child, we learn to control our basic human functions – to stand, walk, talk, feed ourselves, coordinate hand and eye, and control bowel and bladder, thus forming the third layer. The outside layer contains all our cognition, knowledge, abstract thinking and finer skills, which develop over a long time, and this outermost layer is largely what the world sees, values and believes is our 'self'. But dementia attacks our selfhood from the outside, shooting holes in the top two layers until they crumble away, leaving the sensory, emotional, psychological and spiritual elements – our inner self – more exposed and therefore more important. Yet these are often the most neglected aspects of care, particularly in institutional care. Do they give us a clue as to how communication can be made without words?

So, when all Malcolm's outermost layer, together with nearly all his physical functions were crumbling away, including words, we tried to communicate

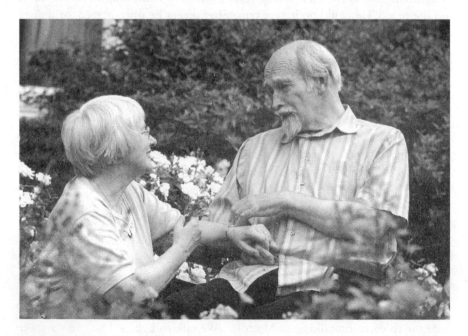

Barbara and Malcolm, 2000

with Malcolm through his five senses: smiley faces, bright colours, changes of viewpoint; the smell of cooking and aromatherapy sessions; the sound of music (recorded or live – even someone humming) and of human voices and laughter. We continued to feed Malcolm orally, however long it took, to give him the pleasure of taste (and social interaction) right to the end. Perhaps the most important sense was touch, especially to help him feel safe: we stroked Malcolm's hands and face, gave him spontaneous hugs and a goodnight kiss. When he sometimes woke in fear in the middle of the night, we didn't run to the medicine bottle, but held him close, whispered in his ear and he would relax and drift off to sleep again. In those ways we were not only communicating with him, we were also trying to meet his most basic spiritual need – to feel loved and cherished.

In his last chest infection, Malcolm gave us clear physical signs that he was world-weary and wanting to let go. His swallowing stopped altogether and he drifted in and out of consciousness. A week later, Malcolm was dying peacefully, surrounded by his close family – including the young grandchildren, who were not a bit fazed. My yoga teacher had recommended that I put my fingers in the little hollow at the nape of his neck and talk to him, while each of us, in a circle, cradled him by holding a part of his body: she said that this was how Malcolm would have arrived in the world, held safely by the midwife, and it would ease his exit. She was absolutely right. The breathing gradually eased, slowed down and finally stopped. We hugged each other in the silence, through our tears.

It had been snowing. Two minutes afterwards, the five-year-old piped up, 'Daddy, can we make a snowman now?' A wonderful reminder that life and death are intertwined.

In the last weeks of his life, Malcolm and I spent a lot of time holding hands and listening to music, especially Stanford's wonderfully evocative choral piece, 'The Blue Bird', which tells the story of someone on a high hill, looking down over a lake, as blue as the sky, over which a blue bird flies, its image held for a moment reflected in the water, before it disappears into the distance. At Malcolm's simple multi-faith funeral, held in his room at our house, I spoke about how I had always thought of Malcolm and his illness as a bird imprisoned in a cage, and that only death could spring the catch and give him a gateway to freedom. So while we listened to the music of 'The Blue Bird', I said I would open the patio door as a symbol of his spirit's flight to freedom. It was a cold day in February, yet as soon as I had opened the door, a bird alighted in the tree outside and sang its heart out until the music finished, then flew into the distance.

Communication is much more than just words.

29

The End of the Story

Tim Dartington

It should not be so difficult to die at home. I suspect that it is what a lot of people want for themselves. My wife Anna was 54 when she got the diagnosis. She talked to a young psychologist about having Alzheimer's disease, about what she called 'my unfaithful brain', and made her wishes very clear: 'I want my husband to be with me and I want to be at home... I am adamant that I want to die at home and not in hospital.'[1]

Anna had been many things in her life. She trained as a nurse and then as a social worker. She worked in a psychiatric hospital and then trained again as a psychotherapist and worked with adolescents and their families. She was a brilliant stepmother to my sons after their mother died. She took a degree in English literature with the Open University. She was going to take a further degree, when she began to struggle with the ordinary things of life, unable to hold things in mind, becoming disorientated, having difficulty walking down steps. For two years she tried to keep going, until the tests showed that something was seriously wrong. A biopsy confirmed that she had Alzheimer's.

She took early retirement and stayed at home with increasing amounts of 'social care'. As her husband, I learned a lot over the next six years about life, about identity and love: I got into training for the patience and perseverance required by doing things I had never done before, like running the London marathon, and I sat in Buddhist meditation as a way of keeping calm.

When Anna was working, she had employed a cleaner, Lynn, who now became her best friend, coming three days a week, not doing much cleaning but sitting with Anna, chatting and laughing. Careworkers from the local authority were coming every morning and evening. There was a no-nonsense Glaswegian; also a Ugandan Asian in her elegant hijab. We employed several young women from Poland to be with Anna during the day.

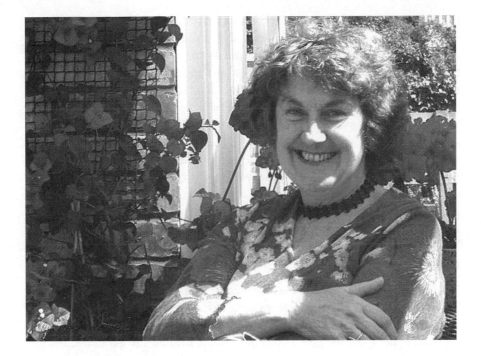

Anna Dartington

We had a volunteer from Age Concern who also became a very good friend. She had spiky red hair and snaky tattoos up her arms, and while Anna could still walk, they would go shopping for outrageous clothes. But later, Anna threw a paperweight at another volunteer. Evening care was difficult at times, and we had three or four different people coming in the week. Anna would be unhappy with a new face. Even the best had to ask questions, which frustrated her, and some did not bother to ask, which was worse. Those that found it too difficult stopped coming. One of the Polish women, Joanna, kept on coming over three years, and by the time we are now talking of, we had a good team of people who knew Anna and she knew them. There were always going to be crises when any one of them was away for any reason, but generally speaking, we had a care system in place – one that Anna could live with.

Her friends, mostly women, continued to visit. She liked to flirt with men friends, but they did not come to see her so often. And increasingly, the visitors were finding it distressing. She might not recognise them or she remembered and started to cry.

I was not always calm of course. I did not see myself as the carer. They talk of support for the carer when they have run out of ideas for the person herself – but the best support for me was that she got the help she needed. So I saw myself more as her protector and perhaps the manager of the care she was getting. I got tired and angry, and at times I saw myself as coping or non-coping with the stress of caring, and as being active or passive in relation to the challenges: on one axis, saint and sinner, and on the other, hero and martyr. As saint, I have a sense that I am doing the right thing; but as sinner, that I am not up to the challenge. As hero, I have a sense that I am making a difference; as martyr, though, I am resigned to my fate. The comments of others would reinforce these states of mind. 'I admire your courage': I was definitely heroic! 'I don't know how you do it': martyrdom awaits.

Then, when I was feeling more of a martyr than a hero, our lives changed again. Anna was assessed for NHS continuing care – by now she was very dependent on care for everything – and we had someone to live in.

I was writing a blog at the time, to counter the isolation I felt, and to record what was happening with Anna:

> And why, when we have a carer living in now, does she immediately look so much more now like someone in an institution? I do not think that it is a coincidence that just in these few days she seems to be giving away a big slice of her independence. I asked the carer if she had any questions. Yes, she said, she could not get the remote to work for the television.[2]

It was like having a landlady in the house. Also, the carers from the different systems, from the agency who provided the live-in care, from the local authority, and those we employed directly, did not always get on. Sometimes there was a sullen stand-off or occasional shouting matches. Their differences emerged in arguments about how to lift Anna, and spread to other aspects of the care: how to feed Anna, talk to her, give her support, and so on. Perhaps we should expect these tensions – the intransigence of the illness can make anyone defensive of their competence.

But I remember it all now as a kind of golden time. This must sound daft. But the uncertainties, the panics, the emergencies, were now under control, I felt, and we had a system that was rigorous enough to cope with whatever Anna's illness threw at us. And what I miss now is the sense of community that developed around Anna to counter the isolation of her illness.

We had the advantages of living in a multicultural society, and, I realised, a global market in care. One live-in carer was a Pentecostal Christian from Sierra Leone, a widow with five grown up children. Another was a Muslim from Kenya, training as a medical student in Turkey, wanting to work in the USA, and paying for it by working as a carer in the UK.

We had a good Christmas, our twenty-first together in this house. I bought a Christmas tree as tall as Anna. My sons stayed over and the live-in carer at the time was another young woman from Eastern Europe who brought a lot of her energy into the household. Anna was also in good spirits, responding much better to sounds than sights: she was very funny about the Queen's speech, though she could not recognise the Christmas tree.

I was away for a week in the spring, and when I got back, I saw little difference in Anna at first. Anna's difficulties on the stairs had always been a focus of our anxiety. Coming downstairs took her twenty minutes sometimes, getting to thirty. She would have a look of intense concentration, and some-times of reverie. She would stop for several minutes, and sometimes she sat down, a test of nerve for anyone who was with her. Any attempt to pressure her was counterproductive. You saw her struggle, put a foot forward, take it back, do this a dozen times, twenty – but taking hold of her physically to help her was as likely to have her slump down on the stair, an immovable object.

Then, one evening, Anna could not get up the stairs at all. For half an hour we stood, her, the carer, me, but she never even got to put her foot on the first step. For months the going up and down the stairs had been a strug-gle, a residual holding of her independence, keeping her frail frame on the move. But now she had stopped, full stop. So I lifted her and the carer took her legs and somehow I got her to the top of the stairs, though I was fearful of dropping her. I was not going to be doing that again.

Next day her friend Lynn was distressed: 'Is she going to die?'

Anna sat in what had been her mother's chair, a traditional straight back, with wings to catch her lolling head, but she kept slipping forward, almost flat out. Then she sat up but she also got up, standing, wavering, uncertain what to do next, turning, questioning, falling back in the chair – except when she fell to the floor.

We needed a better chair, there and then. We would need it perhaps for a week or two, a month or three, it was hard to know. Social services struggled to keep up with her needs. Their assessments were always static, what she needed at that time – which would then take some weeks to get authorised and supplied – and by then her needs would have changed again. A year before, they had ramped the front path, but the process took eight months and by then Anna did not want to go out. And it was not their policy to approve a recliner chair for someone who had already been provided with a state-of-the-art hydraulic bed.

So we were having a nerve-wracking time. Turn your back for a few sec-onds and Anna might fall. It was difficult to maintain such a level of surveil-lance through the day.

I sat with Anna one afternoon, while she lay distressed: she was flapping in the bed, like a turtle on its back. Suddenly, after an hour, she spoke clearly:

'I don't want to go away.' I said she was not going anywhere, she was staying there. Then she relaxed.

One day, she was standing and sitting, standing and sitting all afternoon, and it looked as if she wanted to walk. She was making word-like sounds though it was not possible to understand her, mostly. Then, with the new medication she was taking to calm her agitation she became quiet and hardly talked at all.

I remembered an earlier conversation, when Anna was saying, 'I'm frightened now. But I know you will be with me. I get very low.'

And I said, 'It's understandable.'

'You think so? That's a nice thing to say.' She knocked over a glass. 'It's not juice I want, it's love. Come back.'

'I'm here,' I said. (But I was not really. I was with my own thoughts and she realised, quick enough. Having Alzheimer's didn't mean that she had lost all insight. She could not see a glass in front of her but she knew if I was listening or not.)

So she said, 'Come back. The real you. You were a lovely man. Not now.'

'I thought you might have a drink with me.'

'No! After you have been so horrible to me, I'm afraid I can't. How can you do this? After all the things I did for you.'

Now she slept or was half-asleep all day, eyes closed. Sometimes she seemed to try to get up but could do little except raise her legs. Her body and limbs stiffened, with small convulsions, her left arm twisted, and she bent forward and to the side. Mostly, though, she was quiet and still. By now I would not know if she recognised my voice.

The live-in carer was suggesting that Anna might stay in bed for a time during the day, to ease her soreness. I was not sure about the logic of that, but I had to accept that she looked more passive and potentially bed-bound. The carer also wanted to shave her pubic hair. She said they did that in residential care. I thought, that's another good reason for her not to go into residential care.

And then, on a bright Sunday morning, two carers were getting her up and Anna was having difficulty with her breathing, which was noisy and an effort. Also, she would not open her eyes, respond in any way. The carers wanted me to call the doctor, but the out-of-hours services interrupted me as soon as I mentioned breathing difficulties, before I could explain the context, and told me to call the emergency services. Thirty minutes later Anna was in the accident and emergency ward. It all happened very quickly and without any discussion.

They put in a drip, took blood for tests, and I just managed to stop them inserting a catheter to take a urine sample. I explained about the care we had at home and persuaded the doctor to let her go. But it was hard work, as they wanted to admit her for observation. When Anna cried out the doctor appeared again, worried that she was in pain. In fact, she was making her own protest and after six hours I got her home, but it was a close run thing.

The next Sunday, Anna looked fine with the carers and I was going out. But I came back from the car to get my coat, and found them calling out, 'Where's the telephone? Call 999!' The carers thought that Anna was having a fit, or perhaps a stroke. She was breathing heavily, there was blood on her mouth, and she was thrashing around.

Again, I had no choice but to call the emergency services. The paramedics gave Anna oxygen, and took her blood pressure and temperature. Anna by now had her eyes open, and was agitated. They were saying she would have to go to hospital. I asked why. Because of the tests: she might have cerebral bleeding. So what could they do then? I asked. I said it was important for her to be comfortable and explained that we had a kind of hospital at home, with the bed, the two carers.

They said, 'Is this how she is usually?' and I was saying yes, but the carer was saying no. Anna was agitated, but her breathing was returning to normal. There was no more bleeding from the mouth. I said I did not want her to go to hospital, but they said that this was their advice. They said they would call their supervisor.

Anna was somewhat agitated – which I saw as a good sign. There was not too much wrong if she could protest as she did, with an oxygen mask on her face and a room full of people in green.

I found the discharge letter from A & E the previous week and they were able to compare test results. The paramedics' supervisor arrived. Happily, Anna's breathing was now normal. They took away the oxygen and she was still able to breathe all right. The supervisor explained again that it was their advice for Anna to go to hospital and he asked that I sign a form saying that I had rejected this advice. He said that I should call the doctor, so I did, but the out-of-hours service questioned why I needed a doctor if I already had the emergency services. I gave the phone to the paramedics to sort this one out.

This was our dilemma: 'out of hours', there was nothing between making Anna comfortable as best we could and getting the flashing blue light treatment. When the doctor did come, she was very sympathetic and helpful, and reassured us that we had done the right thing. Anna was comfortable and sleepy by this time. She examined Anna's chest and heart, noted that she had a slight fever. She even attempted a urine sample from the continence pad that the carers had disposed of – less invasive than inserting a catheter.

Anna rested in bed until lunchtime, when the carers got her up. We were back to normal. But if I had not returned for my coat, because I was feeling the cold, she would again have gone to hospital, would have been admitted and, I suspect, would have died in hospital.

And so we managed to hold the line – just – before the next review meeting. I was asked if I would draft what I wanted to see in an advance care plan, having had it explained what this was. I remember thinking, 'But isn't that your job? You are the professionals,' but then realised that I was being taken seriously, treated as an equal in the system. We were responding to an emergency, and were working it out as we went along.

There was someone new to me at the review meeting: the consultant doctor from the palliative care team. The last pieces of the jigsaw of care were now fitting into place and the advance care plan was agreed: to care for Anna at home without any heroic interventions to prolong her life, with copies to the GP, social services, district nurses, the live-in carers' agency.

The palliative care consultant visited us at home, and we had all the back-up we needed now, including different medications just in case, and an oxygen cylinder.

Sometimes Anna got agitated and there was not much we could do to get her comfortable. She wanted to stand up, but did not have the strength. Although she was weak, she could hold my hand in a fierce grip. I had to accept that she was dying, but it was not at all certain how long it would take.

So we had a quiet time over the Easter weekend. I would sit with Anna at times and otherwise have a rest. Our Polish carer told me how on Saturday she and her boyfriend would go to the Polish church with their food in a basket, to be blessed. The evening carer did not come, but we coped some-how. I watched the television news: there was another teenage killing, a boy knifed in a neighbouring London borough. Then I watched the golf, the Masters from Atlanta. Watching other people being skilful is always encour-aging – one less thing I have to be good at.

Two old friends, who had known Anna since school days, came round to see Anna on a surprise visit. It was unusual because mostly her male friends had stopped seeing her when she became ill. I gave them a drink and took them upstairs to see her. Mike sat and held her hand. Derek just stood. He said afterwards that he had not expected the illness to affect her so physically. I explained how she was wasting away, that I thought she would die in the next few months. I said months, but meant weeks. We sat in the garden and I told them what had been happening, the crises and now the palliative care. We talked about the old days.

The evening carer came in, looking, I thought, especially beautiful. She had been that day to see the body of her nephew. He was the boy who had been knifed, that I had heard about on the television news. I thought how many carers have their own very difficult lives as first generation or new immigrants, and how we are dependent on them.

I went away to Ireland for a few days – these work trips an attempt to stay with one foot in the world. When I got home, I knew that we were lurching towards the end. I had picked up a heavy cold on the flight back and worried that I would give Anna the cold and that could finish her.

The psychiatrist visited and saw that Anna was struggling, with increased spasms and difficulty of breathing. She seemed visibly upset by the deterioration, as she did at each visit. I was thinking how this must be a stressful aspect of her job: did she ever see anyone doing other than get worse?

It was strange to think that someone as gregarious as Anna had hardly any family and I decided that it was time to write to her cousins. In my head I began to plan for her funeral.

I called the GP surgery but our doctor was away. Another doctor came: 'Is it your mother?' he said. I hated him at that moment.

It was altogether a busy day. There was a changeover of live-in carers. The last piece of equipment arrived: a headrest to fit on Anna's shower chair. We were all set up now, and now that we had all the gear, she was going to die. I was thinking that it might be very soon. Or might she be able to stay as she was for weeks yet? (Or months, I said, even to myself.)

The palliative care consultant visited again with her team. This was the third doctor in as many days, which was a way of judging the seriousness of the situation.

On the Friday afternoon, the Polish carer, Joanna, who had come to us more than three years earlier, when Anna could still have a laugh and sing and dance, was worried about Anna's breathing, which was short and full of effort. We sat with her until she stopped breathing.

The palliative care consultant called after work and wrote out the death certificate. Some of the carers and my family came round, and we had an impromptu wake and sat with Anna during the night. The undertakers took away the body the next day.

The doctor gave the cause of death on the certificate as dementia – which was true enough. Strangely, the coroner's office would not accept so straightforward an explanation and a new certificate had to be issued. Even in death there was a wish to find another explanation for what had been happening.[3]

Notes

1   Anna's account was later published as: Dartington, A. and Pratt, R. (2007) 'My Unfaithful Brain – a Journey into Alzheimer's Disease.' In R. Davenhill (ed) *Looking into Later Life: A Psychoanalytic Approach to Depression and Dementia in Old Age.* London: Karnac, pp.283–297.

2   Tim Dartington's blog can be found at http://dementiathoughts.blogspot.com. Later, Tim used his blog as a basis for his account of his experiences as Anna became more ill, published in the journal *Dementia.* Dartington, T. (2007) 'Two days in December.' *Dementia 6,* 3, 327–341.

3   Tim Dartington has also written about the last few months of Anna's life, with input from the clinical team who cared for her at this stage in her illness, in the *British Medical Journal*: Dartington, T. (2008) 'Dying from dementia – a patient's journey.' *BMJ 337,* 7675, 931–933.

State of Grace

Rosemary Clarke

I was 51, working full-time as a psychotherapist and living on my own, when my mother became more obviously forgetful and confused. I could describe myself in many ways, but 'conscientious' would always be near the top of the list. Now that taking care of my mother became a more evident responsibility, I tried my very best here too.

It would be simplistic to say I had a good relationship with her: things are rarely that uncomplicated. I knew her heart was in the right place, and she was a kind, non-judgemental and compassionate woman, of whom I was very fond. Equally at times I found her profoundly irritating. What is unambiguously true is that for a very long time I had 'taken care' of her. She had very little confidence: she had learned early on to be uncertain of her welcome, and she carried that sense with her all her life. I understood her difficulties and had always tried to help her through them, to 'make things better', as far as possible. I would include her sometimes in social events of mine; when she needed new clothes, it was I who would accompany her and encourage her; I went with her to medical appointments. Mother–daughter roles reversed, in part at least, from way back. And of course we were not unusual in this. So many women slip into being carers without noticing it. I no more thought of myself as a 'carer' at the end of 1998 than as a spacewoman.

When I began to be concerned about the level of my mother's functioning, my brother's view was more relaxed. He thought she didn't remember which day of the week it was because she didn't go out much: one day was pretty much like another for her, he reasoned. But then, my impression was that his attitude generally was not to look beneath the surface of things. I remember going with her to the consultant who was to perform her hip replacement operation and having to supply most of the information. And there was more than simple forgetfulness: I recall that she was uncharacteristically 'selfish' about wanting to go ahead immediately with the operation, whatever the effect on others. I was about to move house but, unusually, that didn't seem to affect my mother's wishes.

I know now that my biggest difficulty was not her illness itself, not our pre-existing relationship, not even my limited time, but the fact that I knew nothing about dementia. I didn't even know the word and, worse still, simply thought she was 'going senile' as her mother had done, and that we just had to do the best we could. The district nurse from her GP practice didn't mention the word, didn't mention diagnosis, didn't mention memory clinics or drugs for dementia, or the Alzheimer's Society or support groups or respite care, or… I could go on. I often do! As far as I knew, I just had to get on with it and do the best I could, and we lurched together into what became a kind of awful chaos.

It was after she had the lengthy anaesthesia for the operation a few weeks later that she went deeply into dementia: she was hallucinating wildly and was very paranoid. On her return from hospital she made life impossible for the live-in carer we had employed. She refused to do any of her exercises, and would only do anything if one of us was there. Things went from bad to worse; she fell and dislocated her new hip joint no less than three times, and after three emergency trips to hospital she had to have the whole thing re-done, with another long period of anaesthesia. I was sitting by her bed when she asked me what the children were doing on the floor over there. It was probably a couple of years later, and after many such comments – also including mention of dogs she was seeing – that I heard of dementia with Lewy bodies, and put two and two together.

Several months elapsed, during which my mother's condition deteriorated. She lost weight, and clearly was only eating when someone was there. The morning I came in and found her vest draped over her bedside light with a brown-rimmed hole where it had burned through is etched in my memory, as is the occasion when she rang me 40 times in one day.

The other thing that was happening – apart from my brother and me running to keep up with her, and me tearing my hair out metaphorically, dashing between my appointments to find out if she was all right as she'd not answered the phone, all the while trying to set up caring arrangements which she always sabotaged – was that we were visiting what seemed like all the residential care homes in the area. And none was any good, as far as she was concerned. 'Frazzled' is too easy a word for how I felt during this time. I was near my wits' end, frustrated that she was being so 'difficult', and not understanding that she really couldn't help herself.

In the end we conned her – that is the truth – into going into a nursing home for the daytimes, and I felt the most colossal relief when I left her that morning. Thank God someone was looking after her for the day, and I could stop worrying for a few hours.

After a while, my mother moved into the home; she stayed there for some years, and gradually her mental and then her motor faculties deteriorated. Eventually, I somehow found my way to the Alzheimer's Society, and found the enormous relief of being with others in the same boat, who understood. A wonderful community psychiatric nurse, who was the carer support worker, introduced to me to all sorts of information and I gradually began to get the picture. But time after time I would discover something just too late for it to be useful for my mother. She had, for example, 'become incontinent' before I learned that much so-called incontinence in dementia is more to do with the person not remembering where the loo is, or with needing help to remember to go at regular intervals, than about loss of bladder control.

The hardest thing for me was, and still is, that I was unable to provide her with a decent quality of life, at a time when she was utterly dependent on those around her to do so – and when, moreover, that quality of life was possible, if I and others had known what we did not know. I don't blame myself. I don't even feel guilty, just terribly sad, that what was possible did not happen for her, and that she had some truly awful experiences which need not have happened.

That said, I want to describe some sublimely lovely times we had together, which in some ways were made possible by her greater simplicity and immediacy. While I could still get her into the car, we went out together at weekends. I can remember sitting with her in the garden room of my house, with the autumn sun coming weakly through the glass, as we sorted the apples from my orchard: perfect ones for keeping, in that box, those with a slight blemish into this one, and into the bowl the ones needing to be prepared and frozen straight away. Of course, she asked me again every time she picked up an apple what the categories were, but it didn't matter. She was perfectly content, in a garden, with her daughter, and being useful. And I could feel I was giving her what she needed.

One summer afternoon, I drove her to a tiny village where we parked the car and made our way, very slowly, along a track then down to a stream. I unfolded the chairs I'd somehow managed to carry with my spare hand and sat her down, and we spent a memorably content couple of hours just being together. A swan glided along, birds sang, the sun warmed her old bones, and we even had a little picnic, magicked from my rucksack. It was the sort of place we each loved, it was just right for her, and it was a chance for me to be still and peaceful for a while in my very full life.

I took my mother several times to the Sunday afternoon concerts at the Barber Institute in Birmingham. It was liberating for me that whatever my mother did, I knew I would not be embarrassed by her. She could clap her appreciation after each movement if she wanted to. Why ever not? When you have little time left to enjoy beauty, social conventions become unimportant.

Tiny simple things became significant and precious. We would pass a house with a lavender bush at the front, and I would squeeze a bit and offer my fingers to her to sniff. The smile that came over her face as she tried to say she remembered and loved that smell was so rewarding.

But back at the nursing home, she had, I was told, become 'aggressive'. At the time I knew nothing of what this might signify – pain, fear, an attempt to communicate something really important. So, when the nursing home asked my permission to sedate her, I reluctantly agreed. I didn't realise they meant permanently. I didn't know that she had a Lewy body dementia, nor that such drugs can be fatal to someone with that illness. There was absolutely no culture of partnership in the management of the home, and I always ended up feeling a nuisance when I asked to discuss things with the staff. So, although I spent that Christmas lunch more or less lifting my mother's head out of her food because she was so drowsy – I do not exaggerate – somehow, it was only some weeks later, when she was still 'out of it' and I enquired if it might per- haps be a result of the sedative, that I discovered that she was still being given this stuff and that 'it took a while to get the dose right'. I was horrified!

Shortly after this, no surprise, Mummy had a fall, broke her femur, was hospitalised, was not operated on because of the previous difficulties with the anaesthesia, and was discharged, against my express wishes, back to the same nursing home. I demanded that the psychogeriatrician see my mother, and thank heavens he ruled that she should not be given the drugs any more. There followed a lengthy period in which the diary we kept shows my mother apparently 'absent' for much of the time, not responding to me, not seeming to recognise me, just 'vacant', eyes either closed or open but not seeing. As it seemed. No matter what I tried, there was no response.

For some time I had been managing my mother's finances, and I found that a struggle emotionally. Previously, my brother had been carrying out this task, but without consulting me or getting me to sign cheques, even though I was joint attorney with him. Our relationship had been poor for many years – ancient history that continued to bedevil our dealings with one another. A lack of trust on my part finally spilled over into outright anger, whereupon he handed all the papers to me. At this stage, I was only just keeping my own head above water financially. It was not appropriate for me to be taking on new patients at a time when I was so distracted; consequently my income was slowly but surely diminishing to the point where I didn't buy even a cup of tea for myself if I went out, and was praying that my car wouldn't need replacing or the roof spring a leak. There were simply no reserves.

Yet here I was now, co-signing my mother's cheques for £2000 every month to pay the nursing home. I felt a kind of impotent rage that the state expects people with dementia to pay for their own care, unlike people with other terminal illnesses, and that I had to fight decisions even about the paltry so-called 'nursing care' contribution, and any other little benefits to which she was supposedly entitled.

But among all this exhaustion and distress and frustration, two very important things happened, both of which were a huge relief, and brought great blessings.

One of the big changes was that we found another, quite different, nursing home for the final year of my mother's life. The keypad on the front door meant that I could pop in any time, as though this was my mother's home, which of course it was. From the start, I was there as a partner in her care, accepted and valued as such, and felt completely free to speak with the sister or the manager. Mostly, I had the delightful experience of being able to affirm the very good care the staff provided. When something was not right, my criticisms were accepted just as easily. The staff asked me to complete a form including an account of my mother's life story, so that they knew something about her even though she could not tell them herself: she was now silent and nearly always apparently unresponsive when spoken to. Sometimes a member of staff and I would hug each other when I arrived. Many were East European women, far from their families, and I was losing my mother. Real human warmth existed between us.

I'm remembering her ninety-first birthday, a few days after she arrived. A Sunday afternoon; her room is filled with flowers. Some staff and some kind friends of mine are gathered there and we are all drinking champagne cocktail, a drink she'd always loved. Mummy's face is not so unresponsive now: it is clear she is enjoying hers. And the cook brings in a magnificent cake and we all sing 'Happy Birthday', for the last time as it will turn out. Such events were rare, of course, but I felt happy, knowing I was doing the best I could for this dear woman, and that she was, perhaps, happy too.

The second of these late gifts was that a colleague told me about a course in 'coma work', which was said to benefit people in 'withdrawn' states such as coma or dementia.[1] I felt doubtful that it could help my mother. Was she not *unable* rather than withdrawn? But I had to give it a try, so I went on the course. From what I heard that weekend, I could appreciate that this method had helped many other people, in quite dramatic ways, but I left feeling fairly neutral about it. What I took away was the very simple notion that I needed to look for any signs of activity from my mother and support her to express those to their fullest; that my task was to enable *her* expression rather than to try to express myself to her. That was the radical change of mindset that took place within me.

At the time I began to try this method with my mother, she had not spoken to me for a year. Her open eyes seemed to see nothing outside herself. She habitually lay with her arms crossed across her chest, her hands in fists, and with her legs crossed, almost motionless. I assumed she didn't recognise me any more. Yet now, when I really paid attention, I saw anew the tiny movements I'd noticed but not given value to: she would chew her gums, her thumb would wiggle inside the fist, and sometimes a toe would move.

The first time I visited my mother after the course, I tried out what I had learned. The effects were startling. I knelt by her reclining chair and spoke to her: I told her I was going to put my finger on her wrist. I watched her tiny signs of activity and chose to go with the thumb imprisoned within her fist. I put my index finger on the heel of the thumb, which was all I could reach, and 'spoke' with the thumb while also saying how energetic it was, how it seemed to be busy in there. From that simple beginning there flowed 40 minutes of non-stop activity on my mother's part. It was not long before her arm was waving around in the air, my finger always staying gently but firmly attached to her hand. She made sounds, then she spoke, at first odd words, then short sentences. All the while I was encouraging her to do whatever it seemed her body wanted to do, both with my words and their tone.

When I was leaving, I said, 'Goodbye for now,' and she replied, 'Goodbye for now,' and, after a little pause, 'You *are* kind, darling.' I will never forget that moment: it took my breath away.

Over the next five or six months, we nearly always had some form of connection when I spent time with her. When she didn't make any response, that was easier because she seemed to be *choosing* to ignore me. To choose, even to reject, in a life of almost total passivity seemed to me valuable. As well as the obvious benefit to my mother, this process was a gift also to me: I let go of needing to 'understand' and learned instead to trust my intuitive responses. It may seem strange, but I am in many ways grateful to this illness for giving Mummy and me a way to connect more closely than we probably had since I was a baby.

She chose to use the coma work with me for about six months, and then

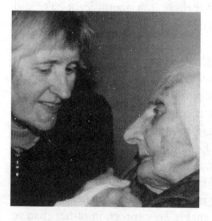

Rosemary with her mother Josan

she 'went inside' again for almost a year. Finally, with the crisis of leaving this world to face, she chose to take it up again.

She 'announced' one December day that she was dying, by refusing food and even liquid. She had shut her mouth against food before, but this was different: she didn't begin to eat again after a while as she had done previously. I had been due to go away for a week, but it was simple to cancel my holiday and stay with her instead.

Those last two weeks were little short of miraculous, at least for me. My training, probably as a therapist and certainly in coma work, enabled me to be there for her, always fully present, sometimes silently. The word I would use to describe our connection was communion. We used our respective thumb and finger, with her constantly holding one of my fingers. She did a number of things repeatedly, and I felt able to participate in a way that I believe held her in love, just as we were both being held in love by the staff. One example is particularly vivid. As she lay quite still in her bed, she would quite suddenly and almost abruptly turn her head and look up and away to her left, her eyes wide open, as though seeing something or someone unseen by me, perhaps the oft-quoted bright light, or perhaps people she had known. I was confident in encouraging her to look away from me, here and now, and towards what was to come, both by what I said and by the tone of my voice, and with constant contact with her finger. 'You seem to be seeing...' (and I didn't fill in what or whom, because I didn't know) '...That looks good,' or 'That looks interesting,' or 'exciting'. Then, equally suddenly, she would turn back towards me and grip my finger tightly. Now I would say to her things like, 'You are afraid? I *know* you will be all right.' And there was no bravado in me: I really knew this to be true. At other times when she would turn and grip my finger, I, who had been with her through so much in her life, would say, 'You know, Mummy, this is the one thing you have to do alone: this time I cannot come with you.' And I said it with a very simple love and with complete confidence, a confidence born out of the learning that had come out of all those years of stress and struggle and heartache.

As it was coming up to Christmas, I sang her some of the traditional carols which she had loved. I said prayers of commendation from the old prayer book, prayers which had been familiar to her, and which offer courage and confidence and hope to the dying, prayers which came from another part of my life but which now felt right, and true, and full of meaning.

I took comfort from being able to be with my mother in these ways. Together, I believe, we were floating on a sea of unknowing, of completely trusting. Sometimes I wept quietly, tears of loss but also of letting go. I felt very relaxed, even serene, and at peace in myself. The imminence of her passing was not a worry, but the herald, I somehow knew, of a moving on: for her, to something better, and for me, to a different kind of rest. And I too surrendered now, to 'Whatever Is'. I had arrived at what is perhaps called by religious people a state of grace. In that time I had a sense of what I cannot now describe adequately. I can only say things like: the mystery of being, the possibility of our continuation in some way eternally, a sense of our connectedness one with another, and of being faintly in touch with 'Something' much greater than everything, in which all is held.

My dear mother's dying, set, as it was, within the unobtrusive but profoundly competent and loving care of the nursing home staff, gave me one of the many infinitely precious gifts which came out of my mother's illness.

It may seem strange to speak of the gift of my mother's dementia, and I certainly only refer to it as – in some ways – a gift to *me*. I cannot but believe that for her, much of the time, especially earlier on, it was quite dreadful. But I learned much, especially in the last year or so – about being less cerebral, about what that word grace could mean, about the loving kindness of the nursing home staff. And well before my mother died, I received a heartfelt apology from and reconciliation with my brother. Her illness took me to places in myself to which I might not have gone. The greatest gift was that this experience – my intimate connection with my mother's slow dying – gave me in a way a chance to rehearse my own approach to death, as a traveller with the person dying, as a witness that it can be a serene and peaceful journey, and that it may hold within it 'Something' more.[2]

Notes

[1] More information about coma work can be found in *Coma: a Healing Journey* by Amy Mindell (1999). Portland: Lao Tse Press or at www.aamindell.net, accessed 28 March 2009.

[2] Rosemary Clarke first wrote about her experience of coma work in an article published in the *Journal of Dementia Care*. See Clarke, R. (2004) 'Precious experiences beyond mere words.' *Journal of Dementia Care 12*, 3, 22–23.

Glossary

Alzheimer's disease the most common cause of dementia. An illness which alters the chemistry and structure of the brain, causing brain cells to die. Alzheimer's disease was first identified by the German neurologist Alois Alzheimer in 1906.

Anti-psychotic drugs major tranquillisers or sedatives, also known as neuroleptic drugs. They are sometimes used to sedate people with dementia who are displaying aggressive or restless behaviour. There is concern about the side-effects of these drugs (including drowsiness, dizziness, unsteadiness, reduced mobility and coherence, increased risk of stroke and heart attack), and increasing evidence that they may accelerate the rate of decline in people with dementia, and lead to premature death. For people who have dementia with Lewy bodies, there is strong evidence that anti-psychotic drugs may be particularly dangerous. See Alzheimer's Society *Factsheet 408: Dementia: Drugs used to Relieve Depression and Behavioural Symptoms* (www.alzheimers.org.uk/factsheet/408) and the report of the All-Party Parliamentary Group on Dementia, *Always a Last Resort* (2008), available at www.alzheimers.org.uk/downloads/ALZ_Society_APPG.pdf, accessed 28 March 2009.

Aricept brand name for donepezil, a drug which can be effective in improving symptoms and temporarily slowing the progression of decline in some people with Alzheimer's disease. Currently NICE guidelines recommend its use only for people at a moderately advanced stage of the disease but the Alzheimer's Society is campaigning for it to be prescribed to people at an earlier stage of the illness. See www.alzheimers.org.uk/factsheet/407 and www.alzheimers.org.uk/site/scripts/documents.php?categoryID=200264, both accessed 28 March 2009.

CAT scan (or CT scan) a computerised axial tomography scan, which uses a series of x-rays taken from different angles to build a three-dimensional image of part of the body; a CAT scan of the brain may be used to assist in the diagnosis of a dementing illness.

Continuing care a term often used to refer to long-term nursing care and treatment, managed and fully funded by the NHS; strictly speaking this is called 'NHS continuing healthcare'. NHS continuing healthcare is free to the user, as opposed to so-called 'social care' provided by the local authority, for which a charge is generally made, subject to a means test. The majority of people with dementia receive social care rather than free NHS continuing healthcare.

CSCI the Commission for Social Care Inspection, the public body which used to regulate care homes in England. This body has now been replaced by the Care Quality Commission (CQC).

Dementia a clinical condition which may be caused by a number of different physical diseases of the brain. Dementia is characterised by a progressive decline in cognitive and physical functioning, including memory, concentration, reasoning, understanding and communication skills, and the ability to carry out daily activities independently, such as cooking or getting dressed. More than half of all people with dementia also develop behavioural and psychological symptoms such as depression, delusions, aggression, wandering or loss of inhibitions. The most common types of dementia are Alzheimer's disease and vascular dementia.

Dementia with Lewy bodies (also known as Lewy body dementia) a type of dementia in which abnormal protein deposits, known as Lewy bodies, develop inside nerve cells in the brain, interrupting the brain's normal functioning. A person with this type of dementia typically fluctuates in his or her mental abilities from day to day, and may experience hallucinations. Some symptoms are similar to those of Parkinson's disease, including tremors and slowness of movement.

Early onset dementia (also known as young or younger onset dementia) dementia which develops before the age of 65.

Fronto-temporal dementia a rare form of dementia, caused by damage to the frontal lobe and/or temporal parts of the brain. At an early stage, memory usually remains intact while personality and behaviour – including social skills and the ability to empathise with others – may change radically. Language skills may also become damaged. At a later stage, symptoms are usually similar to those of Alzheimer's disease. Fronto-temporal dementia may develop at any age, but is more likely to affect people under 65.

Haloperidol an anti-psychotic drug.

LGBT lesbian, gay, bisexual and transgender.

Mini mental state examination (MMSE) a series of questions and instructions which are designed to assist in assessing a person's level of cognitive functioning and may be used to reach a possible diagnosis of dementia. The questions are designed to test functions such as short-term memory, ability to name familiar objects, being aware of the current date and the day of the week, recall of personal information such as own address, and so on. The MMSE only gives a rough guide to a person's abilities, and the standard test does not give reliable results for people with learning disabilities, physical disabilities such as deafness or blindness, communication difficulties (for example after a stroke) or those who are not fluent in the language in which the test is administered.

Mini mental state score each question in the mini mental state examination is scored. Correct responses to all questions or instructions attract a score of 30.

With most types of dementia, the more advanced the disease, the lower the score on the MMSE will be.

Multi-infarct dementia a type of vascular dementia. It is caused by a series of small strokes, which interrupt the blood supply to the brain.

Neuroleptic drugs another name for anti-psychotic drugs.

NICE the National Institute for Health and Clinical Excellence. An independent agency providing guidance to the NHS on health promotion and clinical practice, and on the use of new and existing medicines and treatments, including recommendations as to which drugs should be prescribed for certain illnesses and conditions.

Parkinson's disease a progressive disease of the nervous system which affects the ability to coordinate movement. It is characterised by a pronounced tremor, slowness of movement and stiff muscles which may lead to an expressionless face. One in three people with Parkinson's disease go on to develop dementia. The illness was first identified by the London doctor James Parkinson in 1817.

Pick's disease a type of fronto-temporal dementia.

Psychiatrist of the working age a psychiatrist who works with patients aged between 17 and 65, as opposed to an 'old age psychiatrist' or psychogeriatrician who usually works with patients over the age of 65. Expertise in dementing illnesses is more often found amongst old age psychiatrists, and a younger person with dementia (under 65) may be transferred from the care of a psychiatrist of the working age to the care of the old age psychiatry team.

Psychogeriatrician a psychiatrist specialising in the assessment and treatment of elderly people.

Risperidone an anti-psychotic drug.

Sectioning the terms 'sectioning' and 'being sectioned' are commonly used to mean being admitted to a psychiatric hospital under compulsion. The term derives from the various 'sections' of the Mental Health Act 1983 which give the authorities the power to detain someone in a psychiatric hospital against his or her will. Two doctors must agree that the person is 'suffering from a mental disorder of a nature or degree which warrants the detention of the patient in a hospital for assessment or treatment for at least a limited period', either for his or her own protection or for the protection of other people.

Vascular dementia dementia caused by interruptions in the blood supply to the brain, usually following a stroke or a series of small strokes.

Younger onset dementia another name for early onset dementia.

Recommended Reading

Understanding dementia

Introducing Dementia by David Sutcliffe. Age Concern England, London 2001.
Caring for Someone with Dementia by Jane Brotchie. Age Concern England, London, 2003.
At your Fingertips: Dementia – Alzheimer's and other Dementias by Harry Cayton, Nori Graham and
    James Warner. Class Publishing, London (2nd edn), 2004.
And Still the Music Plays: Stories of People with Dementia by Graham Stokes. Hawker Publications,
    London, 2008.

Carers' experiences

Alzheimer: A Journey Together by Federica Caracciolo. Jessica Kingsley Publishers, London,
    2006
Dementia Diary: A Caregiver's Journal by Robert Tell. RTP Press, Michigan, 2006.
Losing Clive to Younger Onset Dementia by Helen Beaumont. Jessica Kingsley Publishers, London,
    2009.
Caring for Kathleen by Margaret T. Fray. BILD Publications, Kidderminster, 2000.

People with dementia in their own words

Living in the Labyrinth: A Personal Journey Through the Maze of Alzheimer's by Diana Friel McGowin.
    Mainsail Press, Cambridge, 1993.
Dancing with Dementia: My Story of Living Positively with Dementia by Christine Bryden. Jessica
    Kingsley Publishers, London, 2005.
You are Words: Dementia Poems by John Killick. Hawker Publications, London (2nd edn), 2008.

Resources from Alzheimer's Society

The Alzheimer's Society website contains a wealth of information about all
aspects of dementia care, including Factsheets on a wide range of subjects. All the
Factsheets may be downloaded at www.alzheimers.org.uk/factsheets. Printed copies

of the Factsheets are available on request from Xcalibre on 01753 535751. Up to six sheets are free; further sheets are 20p each.

The Dementia Knowledge Centre at Alzheimer's Society's headquarters in London holds a large collection of books, periodicals, dvds etc. about all aspects of dementia. See www.alzheimers.org.uk/dementiaknowledgecentre. The Dementia Knowledge Centre is open daily, and visitors are welcome by appointment. Telephone: 0845 130 2545. The Dementia Catalogue, a comprehensive database of dementia-related material, is available to all on the website www.alzheimers.org.uk/dementiacatalogue.

Helpful Organisations

England and across the UK

Admiral Nursing DIRECT
Helpline: 0845 257 9406
www.fordementia.org.uk/what-we-do/
admiral-nurses

Age Concern England
Free Helpline: 0800 00 99 66
www.ageconcern.org.uk

Alzheimer's Society (supports people
affected by all types of dementia, not just
Alzheimer's)
Enquiries: 020 7423 3500
Helpline: 0845 300 0336
www.alzheimers.org.uk

**British Institute of Learning Disabilities
(BILD)**
Enquiries: 01562 723 010
www.bild.org.uk

Care Quality Commission (CQC)
Enquiries: 03000 616161
www.cqc.org.uk

Carers Direct
Free helpline: 0808 802 0202
www.nhs.uk/carersdirect

Carers UK
Enquiries: 020 7378 4999
Carersline: 0808 808 7777
www.carersuk.org

Crossroads – Caring for Carers
Enquiries: 0845 450 0350
www.crossroads.org.uk

**Commission for Social Care Inspection
(CSCI)**
CSCI has now been replaced by the
Care Quality Commission (CQC). See
above

Down's Syndrome Association
Helpline: 0845 230 0372
www.downs-syndrome.org.uk

for dementia
Enquiries: 020 7874 7210
www.fordementia.org.uk

Help the Aged
Enquiries: 020 7278 1114
www.helptheaged.org.uk

Jewish Care
Enquiries: 020 8922 2000
Helpline: 020 8922 2222
www.jewishcare.org

Mencap
Enquiries: 020 7454 0454
Helpline: 0808 808 1111
www.mencap.org.uk

**MIND (National Association for Mental
Health)**
Infoline: 0845 766 0163
www.mind.org.uk

National Council for Palliative Care
Enquiries: 020 7697 1520
www.ncpc.org.uk

NHS Direct
24-hour helpline: 0845 4647
www.nhsdirect.nhs.uk

PALS (Patient Advice and Liaison Service)
To find your nearest PALS office ring
NHS direct on 0845 4647
www.pals.nhs.uk

Parkinson's Disease Society
Enquiries: 020 7931 8080
Helpline: 0808 800 0303
www.parkinsons.org.uk

Pick's Disease Support Group
Enquiries: 0845 458 3208
www.pdsg.org.uk

Uniting Carers for Dementia
Enquiries: 020 7874 7210
www.fordementia.org.uk/what-we-do/
uniting-carers-for-dementia

Northern Ireland

Age Concern Northern Ireland
Enquiries: 02890 245 729
Advice line: 02890 325 055
www.ageconcernni.org

Alzheimer's Society, Northern Ireland
Enquiries: 02890 664 100
www.alzheimers.org.uk

Carers Northern Ireland
Enquiries: 02890 439 843
Carersline: 0808 808 7777
www.carersni.org

Down's Syndrome Association: Northern Ireland Office
Enquiries: 02890 665 260
www.downs-syndrome.org.uk

Help the Aged in Northern Ireland
Enquiries: 02890 230 666
www.helptheaged.org.uk

Mencap Northern Ireland
Enquiries: 02890 691 351
Helpline: 0845 7636 227
www.mencap.org.uk

Regulation and Quality Improvement Authority
Enquiries: 02890 517 500
www.rqia.org.uk

Scotland

Age Concern Scotland and Help the Aged in Scotland
Enquiries: 0845 833 0200
Helpline: 0845 125 9732
www.ageconcernandhelptheaged
scotland.org.uk

Alzheimer Scotland – Action on Dementia
Enquiries: 0131 243 1453
24-hour dementia helpline: 0808 808 3000
www.alzscot.org

Carers Scotland
Enquiries: 0141 221 9141
Carersline: 0808 808 7777
www.carerscotland.org

Down's Syndrome Scotland
Information line: 0131 313 4225
www.dsscotland.org.uk

Enable Scotland (for people with learning disabilities)
Enquiries: 0141 226 4541
www.enable.org.uk

Scottish Commission for the Regulation of Care
Enquiries: 01382 207100
Helpline: 0845 603 0890
www.carecommission.com

Scottish Partnership for Palliative Care
Enquiries: 0131 229 0538
www.palliativecarescotland.org.uk

Wales

Age Concern Cymru and Help the Aged in Wales
Enquiries: 02920 431 555
Free Helpline: 0800 00 99 66
www.accymru.org.uk
www.helptheaged.org.uk

Alzheimer's Society, North Wales
Enquiries: 01248 671 137
www.alzheimers.org.uk

Alzheimer's Society, South Wales
Enquiries: 02920 480 593
www.alzheimers.org.uk

Care and Social Services Inspectorate Wales
Enquiries: 01443 848 450
www.cssiw.org.uk

Carers Wales
Enquiries: 02920 811 370
Carersline: 0808 808 7777
www.carerswales.org

Down's Syndrome Association: Wales Office
Enquiries: 02920 522 511
www.downs-syndrome.org.uk

Mencap Cymru
Enquiries: 02920 747 588
Helpline: 0808 8000 300
www.mencap.org.uk

Republic of Ireland

Alzheimer Society of Ireland
Enquiries: 01 284 6616
Helpline: 1 800 341 341
www.alzheimer.ie

Carers' Association
Enquiries: 057 932 2920
Freephone: 1800 240 724
www.carersireland.com

Down Syndrome Ireland
Enquiries: 01 426 6500
www.downsyndrome.ie

The Contributors

Brian Baylis took care of his friend Timothy for ten years (both in care home and hospital). Brian was for many years a principal lecturer at Huxley College, London. He now lives in Somerset and London where he is involved in various campaigns for LGBT (lesbian, gay, bisexual and transgender) people.

Pat Brown, a college lecturer from Luton, cared for her husband Chris who had early onset Alzheimer's and died in 2007 at the age of 57. Pat had to fight to secure appropriate care for Chris, and she continues to campaign for improved facilities through Uniting Carers for Dementia and the Alzheimer's Society.

Gail Chester is a book historian and community activist (according to her business card, so it must be true). She is also a proud Hackney resident, radical feminist, writer, researcher, carer, Jewish mother of a teenage son, and much else.

Rosemary Clarke is a psychotherapist and writer. She now lives on the Malvern Hills and enjoys walking. Her passion for better dementia care than her mother had has led her to be involved in many contexts, currently as chair of Uniting Carers for Dementia.

Tim Dartington has researched the needs of vulnerable people for many years, including older people in hospitals, in residential care and at home. Then his wife Anna developed early onset dementia and he learned at first-hand about how someone with Alzheimer's may live and die in her own home.

Jennifer Davies lives in Birmingham. She is 46, married and works full-time as a private secretary. Jennifer and her siblings care for their mother Patricia who has Alzheimer's disease and now lives in a care home.

Rachael Dixey spent all her adult life with partner Irene, who developed Alzheimer's in her fifties. Rachael cared for her at home whilst also working, until Irene needed residential care aged 60. Irene is happy, extremely well cared for by the home and still recognises Rachael and her brother Gordon.

Marylyn Duncan is a qualified nurse, who had to give up full-time work in 2004 when her 85-year-old mother came to live with her. Being a nurse in no way prepared her for the journey ahead, as 24-hour caring turned her world upside down, psychologically, physically and socially.

Peggy Fray cared for her sister Kathleen for 40 years. Kathleen had Down's syndrome, and developed severe dementia and epilepsy in later life. Peggy is a trustee of the Down's Syndrome Association and a council member of BILD (British Institute of Learning Disabilities). She was named Campaigner of the Year at the Help the Aged Living Legends awards in 2006.

Pat Hill from Maidstone is the wife of Derrick and visits him daily at the nursing home. She is supported by the local Alzheimer's Society branch and Admiral Nurses. She attends the local church, is a member of the Active Retirement Association (ARA) and goes to Tai Chi.

Andra Houchen, 56, cares for her 71-year-old husband who has fronto-temporal dementia and now lives in a nursing home. She works two days a week for Crossroads as a dementia coordinator. The Houchen family featured in an article about dementia in the *Observer*, 17 February 2008.

Louisa Houchen is a graphic designer, and is the daughter of Andra Houchen (above). Louisa and her sister Amanda were both in their early twenties when their father Anthony developed dementia.

U Hla Htay worked in the shipping industry and trained to be a maritime arbitrator. He has been caring for his wife, who has Alzheimer's, for 13 years with support from their family. He is a member of the Alzheimer's Society Quality Research in Dementia Consumer Network and a consumer reviewer and co-author of a review for the Cochrane Dementia and Cognitive Improvement Group.

Debbie Jackson (not her real name) is from South Africa. Her husband lived in a nursing home for eight years and Debbie remained active in his care until his death in May 2009. A member of the Alzheimer's Society and Uniting Carers for Dementia, she also volunteers with a Jewish Care team providing support for family carers.

Maria Jastrzębska is a Polish-born poet, editor and translator, writing in English. Her recent collections include *Syrena* (Redbeck Press) and *I'll Be Back Before You Know It* (Pighog Press). Her drama *Dementia Diaries* was premiered by Lewes Live Literature in 2009. Both her parents suffered from dementia.

Steve Jeffery is a professor of Human Genetics at St George's University of London. He supported his mother when she developed multi-infarct dementia, and after she went into a nursing home, visited her regularly for six years until she died. He was greatly helped by his family.

Geraldine McCarthy, from Cork, Ireland, has lived in London since 1997. She supported her mother and siblings, in Cork, in the care of her father who had dementia and died in 2006.

Ian McQueen is a composer and teacher. He grew up in Scotland, but has lived in London since the 1970s. His mother still lives in Glasgow.

Sania Malik was born in Pakistan and came to London in 1984. Her husband Hassan developed dementia when their daughters Ayesha, Aliyah and Fariha were aged between two and eight. Hassan died in 2006. Ayesha is now married to Aftab, with two children Mariha and Anzar.

Roger Newman is a 67-year-old retired teacher from Margate, Kent. As a result of caring for his partner David, he co-founded the LGBT (lesbian, gay, bisexual and transgender) Support Group of the Alzheimer's Society. (See www.alzheimers.org.uk/gaycarers) In 2007 Roger was awarded the MBE for his charitable work.

Shirley Nurock cared for her husband (a GP) who developed Alzheimer's in his fifties when their three children were young teenagers. Shirley is involved in many dementia research projects and speaks at national and international conferences on dementia care. She runs a carers' organisation which helps educate medical and clinical psychology students about the impact of dementia on families.

Barbara Pointon and her husband Malcolm both lectured in music at Cambridge until Malcolm was diagnosed with Alzheimer's at the age of 51. Paul Watson chronicled their sixteen-year journey in his film for ITV, *Malcolm and Barbara... Love's Farewell* (2007) and Barbara continues to campaign on behalf of people with dementia and their carers. She was awarded the MBE in 2006.

Helen Robinson trained as a nurse in Belfast, and has lived in Dublin for 50 years. She has four children and six grandchildren. She worked as a bereavement counsellor for some years until her husband Chris became ill, and was active in the Alzheimer's Society of Ireland.

Sheena Sanderson is a young pensioner living in rural England. Her husband Philip, formerly an IT consultant, developed dementia after many years of Parkinson's disease. He died in 2009, after Sheena's chapter was written. Names have been changed.

Maria Smith was born in Florence, Italy. She moved to London in 1955, where she met her partner Lonnie in 1967. For the last eleven years, she has been helping him, at home, through his Alzheimer's. Her poem is dedicated 'to Lonnie, who is facing Alzheimer's with courage and good humour, and with his inimitable style'.

Rosie Smith is 51, a teacher and lives with husband and two teenage sons in rural north Essex. She was unhappy with the care her father received in a nursing home. She currently looks after her 87-year-old mother and is determined that her mum does not go through the same experiences as her dad. Names have been changed.

Jim Swift and his wife Jan were head teachers but their careers came to an abrupt end when Jan was diagnosed with Alzheimer's in 2002. Jim now tries to promote awareness of early onset dementia through membership of Uniting Carers for Dementia and the Alzheimer's Society.

Jenny Thomas lives in London, and her mother Marjorie lived in South Wales. These incidents are taken from Jenny's book *Help, Help* (as yet unpublished), which describes Marjorie's treatment and care when she developed dementia with Lewy bodies. The book explores the experience from the perspectives of both mother and daughter.

Lucy Whitman is a writer, teacher and activist who lives in north London with her teenage son. Lucy and her sister Rosalind took care of their parents when they became frail in later life. Their mother Elizabeth had vascular dementia. www.lucy whitman.com

Anna Young is a psychotherapist living and working in East Sussex. Her husband, Crispian, was diagnosed with fronto-temporal dementia in 2005, and entered a care home in 2007. They were married for 39 years and have five children. Crispian died in April 2009, after Anna's chapter was written.

*W*hat is *for dementia?*

for **dementia**
training ▪ development ▪ admiral nurses

for dementia is a charity which works to improve the quality of life for all people affected by dementia.

The objectives of *for dementia* are to:

- promote and develop admiral nursing, a specialist nursing approach focused on meeting the needs of family carers and people with dementia

- develop learning partnerships and provide high quality training for professionals working with older people, carers and people with dementia

- involve family carers in activities to raise awareness and promote understanding of dementia and carers' needs

- promote best practice in dementia care

- contribute to national and local policy on carers, dementia and older people's care

- influence practice and service development.

There are several interconnected strands to the work of *for dementia*, including Admiral Nurses, *for dementia* training, and Uniting Carers for Dementia.

Admiral nurses are specialist dementia nurses, working in the community, with families, carers and supporters of people with dementia. Their name is derived from the nickname of Joseph Levy CBE BEM, the charity's original benefactor, who had

vascular dementia. He was known by his family as 'Admiral Joe' because of his love of sailing.

Working in partnership with the NHS, *for dementia* now has 60 Admiral nurses in certain localities in the UK, and operates a telephone helpline, Admiral Nursing DIRECT, offering advice and support to people with dementia, family carers and professionals.

Admiral nurses:

- work with family carers as their prime focus

- provide practical advice, emotional support, information and skills

- deliver education and training in dementia care

- provide consultancy to professionals working with people with dementia

- promote best practice in person-centred dementia care.

for dementia **training** aims to improve standards of care for people with dementia and promote good practice by developing the skills and knowledge of careworkers. It provides: a broad range of open courses in London and elsewhere, including courses which provide underpinning knowledge for those working towards NVQs in Health and Social Care; bespoke courses commissioned by organisations and held at their own premises; a certificate programme, *Working with people with dementia and their carers*, accredited by the Open College Network London Region; and training and assessment programmes to assist managers to implement *Skills for Care* standards.

Uniting Carers for Dementia is a network of carers and former carers. Members are committed to using their experiences of caring for someone with dementia to make a difference to the lives of others. Activities include campaigning locally and nationally, contributing to the training and education of professionals, and speaking to the media about what it is like to care for someone with dementia.

Enquiries about any aspect of the work of *for dementia* may be made to:

for dementia
6 Camden High Street
London NW1 0JH
Phone: 020 7874 7210
www.fordementia.org.uk
Registered Charity No. 1039404

Admiral Nursing DIRECT
Helpline: 0845 257 9406